ALZHEIMER'S DISEASE

HELP AND HOPE

Ten Simple Solutions for Caregivers

Jo Huey

Alzheimer's Disease:Help and Hope
Published by **Alzheimer's Institute**

Copyright© 2001 by Jo McDonnell Huey
Limited first Edition, January 2001
Second Edition, April 2008
15th Anniversary Edition, November 2015

For information or to order copies of this book,
contact:

Alzheimer's Institute LLC
www.alzheimersadvocate.com

ISBN: 978-0-9706652-3-2

Edited by: Virginia Vehaskari, PhD

Cover Design: Rick Albertson
www.rickalbertson.net

Published in the United States of America
Printed by Starnet Business Solutions
Mahwah, NJ 07430

Acknowledgment

Special thanks to my editor Dr. Virginia Vehaskari. Without the persistent and consistent assistance this book would never have been completed.

Special thanks to my daughter, Jenae, and son, Jason, for their consistent inspiration and support.

CONTENTS

CONTENTS (Con't.)

INTRODUCTION

This book and the work I do are dedicated to all persons who are assisting in the care and understanding of persons with Alzheimer's Disease (Sometimes referred to as AD). It is designed to provide you with information to improve the quality of life for your loved one with Alzheimer's and for you, the person most dedicated to their well being.

Guilt is NEVER helpful and before you read further you must make a contract with yourself to not feel guilty. You have been doing the best you know how and that makes you a Champion. If you have not been doing things in the manner that I am suggesting then you have new things to try.

Most people have a great deal of difficulty accepting Alzheimer's Disease Symptoms as true symptoms. There are probably a billion reasons for this misunderstanding and the reasons aren't really the issue. The focus needs to be on actually seeing the symptoms as a manifestation of the disease and not as intentional acts.

Alzheimer's Disease is voiced as a terrible and dreadful disease and little jokes are made by almost everyone about memory problems. Memory problems are indeed a serious part of the diagnostic criteria for this disease and thus impact the other symptoms. The relevance of the memory deficit is how it changes the patient's perception of the world and therefore, how the patient reacts to that changed perception. The point for effective interaction with the patient is to understand that they cannot control the disease process any more than anyone can control the symptoms of any disease. With this disease, unlike any other, there is a generally accepted and consistent attempt made demanding that the patient stop having their symptoms - as if they had a choice! For example, we try to jog their memory, correct an inaccurate statement or tell them to STOP asking the same question or to not repeat inappropriate behavior.

Some examples you might hear:

-   "You know your mother has been dead for years. No, you cannot wait for her to eat dinner."
-   "You did not take a bath today and you need to take a bath because we have an appointment with the Doctor. Then we are going to go to lunch with Jane. After lunch we are going to get you a new pair of shoes. Why are you walking off when I am talking to you? We have to go in here and get your bath and we have to hurry."
-   "How can you accuse him of stealing your things after all he has done for us."

- "That doesn't belong to you now give it back."
- "Why would you take those; we didn't pay for them?"
- "You have got to go back to bed and get some sleep. You have been up half the night and why on earth did you empty these drawers? Who is supposed to clean up this mess? I suppose tomorrow you will want to sleep all day and we won't be able to go to Carol's house and help with the children. I am just too tired to deal with this so you have to get in bed and go to sleep right now. We can't continue like this; no one can live this way; we both have got to get some sleep."
- "Do you remember who this is? What did you have for lunch today? Did Mary visit today?"
- "I just told you that we are not going to the bank today, - it is Sunday and the bank is closed. How many times do I have to tell you we are not going to the bank it is Sunday"
- "You can't wear two shirts, you can't pick that up with your hands, you can't go outside it is raining, you can't keep putting things in the wrong place, you can't go home, you are home"

- "You have got to change your clothes, sit down right here and stop walking around. You must keep your clothes on you are in a public restroom. You have got to change your clothes, sit down right here and stop walking around."
- "Now you are going to take a bath because you haven't had one for two weeks and these nice people are here to help us."

In addition one might actually, for the purpose of providing instruction or gathering information, talk about the person as if they are invisible:

- "Did he take his medicine? He didn't spit it out did he? Did she eat anything? She usually won't eat for someone else."

Are any of the scenarios familiar? You may be thinking to yourself that these aren't symptoms of the disease, this is how people with Alzheimer's act and it drives everyone crazy. Yes, that is the point exactly, this is how people with Alzheimer's act and it truly drives everyone crazy. In response to being driven crazy, the caregiver reaction is to demand that they stop the behavior. THE BEHAVIOR CAN'T STOP. A PERSON WITH ALZHEIMER'S DISEASE IS NOT DOING THIS ON PURPOSE - IT IS THEIR DISEASE AND THAT IS WHY EVENTUALLY THEY ALL ACT THIS WAY!

Don't despair; it is not hopeless. We are halfway to the solution when we have just identified the problem. Think of that old adage "Identifying the problem is half the battle." You are halfway to a solution and yes you have been in many a battle. You are also letting GUILT surface and guilt needs to be sent packing - guilt allows bad feelings to "fester" and we are in search of good feelings.

The search for good feelings for both you and the person with Alzheimer's Disease has to be the main area of concentration. The real clue is that they don't understand their symptoms and truly don't know or remember most of what they are doing. You need to learn to accept their behavior as disease symptoms and you can then try to forget what they are doing. Concentrate on what you need to accomplish. By changing your approach you can become very successful, which in turn helps the person with AD become successful and everything improves.

The solution is truly that simple - the application takes understanding, dedication, practice and REST. This book will provide you with understanding, you already have the dedication, or you would have found a way to escape being with this person by now, like most other family and friends, and you have AMPLE opportunity to practice. Most important, the first step is that you both absolutely must find a way to get some rest - that is rest from each other. Rest is important for all caregivers: family, friends and professionals in the field and it is most important for the person with Alzheimer's Disease.

If you are a family or a friend caregiver it is essential that you take care of yourself and that requires having balance in your life. You cannot just give and give and not replenish yourself or you will GIVE OUT! You need to have interests, friends, and leisure time, even time to run errands and most of all REST! You will not be a qualified caregiver if you are exhausted, frustrated, depressed, and ultimately ill. You will not be there to look out for the person with AD if this disease process kills you and it can, not just in spirit but literally.

If you are a professional caregiver, you have got to find ways to train other persons to take ownership and work effectively with persons with dementia. If you work too many hours, you will lose sight of what you are doing and you will burn out. You must take time on a daily basis. Breaks and meals are essential. You must not work too many hours long term. You need to get away. You need to go places and learn new things and share ideas with other creative persons.

Remember, persons with Alzheimer's Disease need to be accepted and loved and appreciated just as they are, not the way they used to be or the way we want them to be. They need to have friends and interests and the opportunity to spend time with persons like themselves. They must feel accepted and acceptable, useful and competent. A person with Alzheimer's Disease needs to be away from the caregiver as much as the caregiver needs time away from them, regardless of how dependent they seem to have become.

Please be certain to leave guilt out of the process. One way to do that is to review how really unacceptable are the symptoms of most diseases. Take vomiting for instance. If someone were ill because they ate or drank too much, no one would ever suggest that they "hold it in" or chastise them for making a mess or smelling things up or ruining their appetite. That is because we know they can't help a symptom of an illness. Another example is bleeding which is truly awful; blood leaves stains and sometimes people bleed because they cut themselves when they are not careful. No one would ever reprimand someone for bleeding, because one knows that it can't be helped, even if it could have been prevented. Take seizures, as another example, they are frightening, disruptive and can result in further injury. However, no one would tell a person having a seizure to get up and stop seizing, because they could split their head open, swallow their tongue, or that their behavior is bothering other people. One would never ask a blind person to read something, nor a finger amputee to play the piano - yet we always ask a person with memory impairment if they remember.

These examples are designed to gently illustrate that most symptoms of other diseases are disruptive and socially unacceptable, however, they are commonly accepted as unavoidable. We need to see Alzheimer's symptoms in the same light.

WHAT YOU ABSOLUTELY NEED TO

UNDERSTAND ABOUT

ALZHEIMER'S DISEASE!

There was an old clichè about calling the doctor and being told to take two aspirins, go to bed and call in the morning. The lesson was about the doctor not having time for you and not wanting to give free advice over the phone. More subtly it was about you not wanting to go wait in the doctor's office and pay for advice. The result had little to do with the doctor. The free advice often worked because something minor was hurting and you were tired, even too tired to go to the doctor's office. If you had eliminated the pain and the fatigue and were still really ill then you would have needed to see the doctor. In this case you would both know that, "two aspirins and bed" would not have worked.

With Alzheimer's Disease it seems that you often don't even get the two aspirin routine. The doctor might say, "The diagnosis is probably Alzheimer's Disease and there isn't much we can do". They can offer a medication that might keep it from getting worse for an unspecified period of time, but not all doctors are aware of all possible medications. The diagnosis is often delivered with grimness and virtually no advice or understanding of what it means to have Alzheimer's Disease. What everyone has been led to believe is that it is grim, horrible and devastating and your lives will be changed dramatically for the worse for years and

1

years to come. This indeed has been the case for many people. However, there is help and there is hope. I do not in any way wish to minimize the effects of this disease for it is a horrible disease that can last for many years. What I am trying to do is provide you with a way to understand the disease and ways to alter your life so you can enjoy your life and time together, in spite of the disease.

When someone is terminally ill with Cancer it is unfortunately a common practice to avoid the person because you don't know what to say and there is nothing you can do. When someone is diagnosed with Alzheimer's Disease it is common to realize that you don't know what it means to have Alzheimer's Disease. If you do know what Alzheimer's Disease means then you can skip on to chapter one. If you are a professional and you hate simple explanations then skip on to chapter one. This is a very simplistic explanation of what to expect when someone has Alzheimer's Disease. This book is designed as a guide for what you can do to help and there is PLENTY THAT YOU CAN DO TO HELP. THIS DISEASE TAKES A LOT OF TIME, UNDERSTANDING AND PATIENCE BUT IT IS NOT IMPOSSIBLE AND IT DOESN'T HAVE TO BE AS DIFFICULT AS YOU MIGHT THINK. IT IS ABOUT CHANGING YOU AND LOOKING AT THINGS IN A DIFFERENT WAY, WHICH FOR ALL HUMANS IS DIFFICULT. THIS ABILITY TO LOOK AT ALZHEIMER'S IN A DIFFERENT WAY IS MORE DIFFICULT FOR SOME THAN FOR OTHERS. BUT ANYONE CAN DO IT!

It is important, for me, to make you aware that in explaining Alzheimer's Disease I am not describing this in medical or scientific terms. I refer to this description as "lay" terms or as some might say "explaining in plain English". Through the years I have tried to come up with analogies and descriptions with which someone can identify to make this disease more understandable. My premise is that with increased understanding of the disease, care becomes easier. The following includes the questions that are asked most often and the explanations I give, which I have been told were most helpful.

Alzheimer's Disease is a regressive degenerative brain disease:

The brain is deteriorating and the memory (information) is being eliminated, in all or part, in the reverse order that it is acquired and stored. A person with Alzheimer's Disease may not be able to acquire any new information at all, or they may just acquire bits and pieces. A way that is helpful to understand how this works is to draw a large dark squiggle on the blackboard. Underneath it put dates starting from 1920 on the left and going to 2008 on the right. Now I want you to think of this as the brain of a person with Alzheimer's Disease. Take a blackboard eraser and start at the right (2008 side) and erase back towards the 1920 side, don't erase everything all the way, but erase the most on the 2008 side. Now look at the spot (brain) on the blackboard. No matter how good your eraser is it doesn't erase every spot uniformly. But in the part where you erased the hardest, most of the mark is gone.

3

This is a very simplistic illustration of how regression in the brain of an Alzheimer's person is working. It is almost impossible to determine how the erasing stops but we do know that the 1920 information will be there the longest (regressive-reverse order it was stored). That is why they don't know if they ate breakfast but second grade is clear. That is why they don't know your name and they are looking for their mother. That is why they are not at home even if they lived in that home for twenty years or they have just been placed in a facility. They can and will have a clear or lucid moment, hour or day depending on how efficient the eraser has been; some of those chalk areas remain even in the 1990's or 2000's. That is why it is not delusions nor is it hallucinations for them to describe things in the 1940's or 1950's as if it were today, in their brain it is the 1940's or 1950's or pieces of each. If we can understand and imagine that we are in that time with them, life will be easier for both of us. It is not strange behavior on either of our parts, but it is responding to and understanding the needs of someone with a regressive brain disease.

Diagnostic procedure:

Officially the only absolute way to determine if it is Alzheimer's Disease is to have a brain biopsy which is usually done at autopsy. However there is as much as 90% accuracy in diagnosis by doing a battery of tests to rule out other disease processes. In order to really be diagnosed with Alzheimer's Disease it is essential to have an extensive exam that includes MRI, PET, etc. This is important to be certain that the person does not have another disease that requires different and specific treatment.

When the Diagnosis is Probable Alzheimer's Disease:

This means the individual has memory impairment not complete memory obliteration. This impairment is most significant in the ability to learn new information or to recall previously learned information. In addition they must have at least one but may have all of the following cognitive disturbances:

Aphasia, is a language disturbance that can be divided into two categories, expressive and receptive. Expressive means they cannot say what they want to say. Speech may come out in mixed up words, or the person may be unable to form words at all. Receptive means that they cannot make sense of what you are saying. They may have one, both, or none of these problems and this can change over time depending on how the disease continues to effect their brain.

Apraxia, is a problem with carrying out movement despite intact motor functions. My understanding of this is that the brain is giving inaccurate signals to the rest of the body and consequently things don't work right. This may result in changes in movement of the body and can be an explanation for why a person with Alzheimer's paces. It is as if the body doesn't know how to stop; though other 'schools of thought' are that pacing is a sign of boredom. It also might explain involuntary movements, stops, starts, shuffles, small steps, rigidity, inability to use eating utensils, etc. Motor dysfunction creates safety issues and can result in falls and injuries.

Agnosia, is an inability to recognize or identify familiar objects. This too can create many problems for functioning in any environment. There are both dignity and safety issues involved. Not being able to differentiate between a telephone and a remote control is embarrassing, describing a table as a plate holder may be amusing (to others), yet confusing ones toothbrush with the safety razor is dangerous.

Executive Functioning Disturbance, such as planning, organizing, sequencing, abstracting is something that seems to be taken for granted. Each function we perform requires many steps and thought processes. If a person with Alzheimer's Disease has disturbance in this area it becomes very difficult to do everyday tasks around the home, and even maintain personal care. It is virtually impossible to carry out more complex tasks like shopping for groceries, cooking a meal, finding your way home, etc.

These things have to be apparent to the degree that they effect their ability to perform in everyday life in order to receive this diagnosis.

Review this criterion and imagine the loss of ability a person with Alzheimer's Disease faces. Imagine what it must feel like to not learn, retain new information, express words, understand words, move around safely, identify familiar objects or even keep track of what you are doing and where you are going. In addition, it only gets worse and just because there aren't problems in some of these areas today doesn't mean there won't be problems in those areas soon. Really think about this, think about it for your own life and you will begin to understand and appreciate the person for what they can do and you need to stop concentrating on what they can no longer accomplish. When working with a person with Alzheimer's Disease it is essential to keep the magnitude of their disease process in mind, not so you can pity them, but so you can accept them for the person they are today. Then go one step further, form a new type of relationship with this person and enjoy each day with them.

Dementia:

Another subject that seems very confusing is this term called dementia. Many people say that the person with whom they are involved doesn't have Alzheimer's Disease they just have Dementia. Dementia though listed as a diagnosis code for insurance purposes, is not really a diagnosis, it is much better described as a symptom. An easy to understand analogy with dementia is vomiting.

Vomiting is something that is universally known, and with the word comes an actual picture of something with which virtually everyone is familiar. The cause for vomiting can be self inflicted (from too much food or drink), a form of wellness (such as in pregnancy), induced by medical treatment (such as radiation or chemotherapy), psychologically induced (anorexia or bulimia) or an actual result of something that is wrong with the gastrointestinal tract. To be even more specific the different types of vomiting could be discussed (projectile, bile, etc.) but that isn't as commonly known. The point is that vomiting evokes a picture of something and the treatment for it is essentially the same regardless of the cause. In addition, regardless of the cause it is accepted as uncontrollable and the person with the symptom is not blamed or mistreated for having it regardless of the mess or inconvenience it creates.

Dementia for all visible and real purposes looks about the same, it is a progressive-regressive pattern that requires the person with it to require assistance with their activities of daily living. The cause for the dementia is the actual diagnosis. Alzheimer's Disease is the leading cause of dementia, with vascular (from strokes) as the second most common cause for dementia. There are many other causes for dementia but they are all in very small percentages. Currently, most dementia's are referred to as Alzheimer's. There are many reasons for this generalization and probably the most common is that when you say Alzheimer's it seems to have become known enough that most people recognize it. If you say dementia or specify such as vascular dementia there tends to be more confusion. The cause of the dementia makes relatively little difference in the treatment. Persons with a degenerating brain, regardless of what is causing the degeneration, need to be accepted as persons with a disease process that is uncontrollable. They need to be treated with the kindness, understanding and positive interventions that minimize the disease process and maximize their quality of life.

WHY I ABSOLUTELY HAD TO FIND AN ANSWER!

I became interested in Alzheimer's before I even knew what it was. I had the good fortune to know an elderly couple, Ike and Tirza, and I don't ever remember them not being an integral part of my life. They lived across the street from me in a small stucco house surrounded by a white picket fence. Rarely did a day go by that I didn't visit them. I would even sneak out to see them when I was sick at home from school. Blizzard days were especially challenging but I would always manage to get to their house. In their eyes I was always ABSOLUTELY PERFECT - I walked on water - and they were equally perfect in my eyes. I took every triumph and tribulation of my life to them and they always took my side. I didn't realize until much later in life what an incredible form of unconditional love those two people provided for me.

I continued to be very close to Ike and Tirza even after my family moved to another town, I graduated from high school, got married and started my own family. However, they soon were unable to visit me any more because Ike couldn't drive. He had been having many problems, which could no longer be denied after he backed his car out of the garage without opening the door first.

Tirza could never leave him alone. He got out one night when she was at a bridge party and fell in a ditch and was missing for several hours. Ike's condition posed special problems for both of them, as Tirza didn't drive and they were 12 miles from the nearest grocery store. She had problems leaving Ike with anyone as he would throw them out of the house or accuse them of stealing.

No one knew what was wrong with him. The doctor said it was probably hardening of the arteries and many believed that Ike had just gotten old, mean, and cantankerous. I knew he was never mean, he was perfect, but I couldn't prove that to anyone else. Tirza did think that he often was being difficult on purpose because of something she had done or not done. I helped as often as I could but I lived 100 miles away, worked full time, and had two toddlers and a husband.

Trying to be a caregiver from a distance was probably some of the more frustrating days of the experience. I felt so helpless. I knew Tirza needed my assistance and I also knew she was not providing me with accurate information and she wasn't complaining because she wanted me to "have my own life".

Fortunately, we moved back to that small town in the summer of 1972 and I was able to spend time with them on a daily basis. I could do anything with Ike including getting him into the car with me so Tirza could go and shop. He loved my children and they thought he was wonderful. He was very patient and kind with them. This helped a great deal but also reinforced to Tirza, the fact that Ike was doing things on purpose to her because he always cooperated with me. I realize in retrospect that it was the unconditional rapport that he and I had always had that made the difference.

Tirza had more difficulty with him but I feel

certain this was because she had changed her approach with him. She was fearful that she wouldn't be able to get him to do things and would approach him in a manner different than she had before he was ill. Consequently, he seemed to react to her fears almost like a "self-fulfilling prophecy". When he wouldn't do what she asked she would become frustrated and feel helpless and she believed he was angry at her by refusing to cooperate. She never really understood this as part of his disease and no one, including me, ever really understood the disease process enough to suggest his reactions were involuntary. I just knew in my heart that he wouldn't do things like that to Tirza if he could avoid it. I do understand now, in retrospect, that he was reacting to her actions. Her actions showed clearly that she did not understand what to do or why or how things were to be done. Hesitation, confusion, anger, and lack of understanding are still some of the greatest problems today, especially with families. Addressing these problems and providing understanding and simple guidelines to primary caregivers is the reason I give in-services and training sessions and the reason for writing this book.

Ike had a massive stroke and as a result was no longer able to stay at home with Tirza. He had walking and balance problems and he was a large man and Tirza was a small woman. This was in 1972 and home health if it was available at all was certainly not available in a small rural town. There were no alternatives in those days and he had to be placed in a nursing home in the closest town. This town was 12 miles from their house. The home had no idea how to manage Ike. All they knew was that he was old, mean and cantankerous and he would hurt the staff. Consequently, they had him tied in a wheelchair in the day and tied in his bed at night. They were afraid of him so no one wanted to care for him. I went there three times a day, untied him, and cleaned him up and fed him. The staff would tell me to stay away from that "old man" or I would get hurt. Those remarks made me very angry but I wouldn't say anything to them. I was in a very bad position because in those days visiting rules were very strict and I wasn't a blood relative. If I broke the rules I wouldn't be allowed to visit. Before I could leave I had to retie him. He would cry and I would cry and I would leave to the sounds of his yelling, "Kid, kid, don't leave me here kid." I would take Tirza to visit whenever I could and even when she was in the room Ike would ask for her but he never recognized her again. She believed until her death that he never forgave her for putting him in the nursing home even though I tried to convince her that wasn't so. But I was unsuccessful.

The reason I got interested in Alzheimer's Disease was because of the deathbed vow I made the day Ike died. It had been six weeks since he had the first stroke when he suddenly had another massive stroke and died during the night. I vowed that one day I would find out what had been wrong with him and I would do something about it. I wanted to do something about the deplorable care, especially being tied up, and the impact on Tirza's life during the whole illness and especially her guilt about putting him in a nursing home. I was frustrated and angry at the entire situation but not at anyone individually. The home did a very good job for other patients. During those times there was little understanding for a condition like Ike's and so it was handled poorly.

I had the opportunity to address my vow thirteen years later. I had been working primarily in the health care field but in the area of Accounting and Data Processing. I had done some research though and decided that Ike probably had this disease called Alzheimer's. On the bulletin board of the large clinic where I worked there was a poster advertising for respite care persons to work for a grant sponsored by a new organization called A.D.R.D.A. (which stood for Alzheimer's Disease and Related Disorders Association) currently known as the Alzheimer's Association. I applied and was accepted for the part-time position. They especially liked persons like me who already had full-time positions because we were available to work evenings and weekends which was the time that families of persons with Alzheimer's really needed respite.

I took two days of vacation and went through their training program. The program, not unlike many training programs today, was much more about company orientation and correctly completing paperwork for the grant project. There was some information about the disease but very little about how to deal with someone with Alzheimer's Disease.

My first assignment was a very tough one, as was explained to me by the staffing coordinator. This particular family had demonstrated need but the agency had been unable to provide a person who was willing to return after the first visit with this particular client. However, she also told me they had many more clients so I didn't have to return to this particular home again, there were plenty of assignments. She was not exaggerating about the difficulty of this assignment. Within a few minutes I realized how little I knew and how unique my rapport had been with Ike. This little lady was difficult and she was very capable of hurting me. However, I was certain that I could figure out how to do a better job. I was sure that I shouldn't take it personally even though when she hit, pushed, pinched and yelled, it really felt very personal. I went back to help with this lady, not because I am a masochist but because I saw the challenge and the need. I wanted to be for this lady what I had been for Ike. I started to figure it out and I practiced and I learned from her for six years (10 hours every Saturday). Much of what I learned developed the list entitled "Absolutely Never" and is also the basis for this book.

The second assignment I received was another little lady and she was difficult in a very different way. She had such intact and refined social skills that it appeared to the untrained eye that there was nothing wrong with her. She lived in a suite in a nursing home and her family hired someone to be with her all the time so she wouldn't be frightened and/or chemically and physically restrained. She loved to wander around the entire home and would ask people to call security because a thief was following her around. The person caring for her was obviously the thief. She did many other things to make working with her very difficult but I saw this as a challenge. Her daughter convinced me to move my family and this lady into a house where I became the primary caregiver. The family paid for someone to be with her 12 hours a day 7 days a week while I went to work and school. I had the responsibility of hiring and training these persons and I had the sole responsibility of her care the other 12 hours a day 7 days a week.

Working effectively with her became a means of survival for me and being able to impart that information to the persons I hired became essential in order to maintain staff to work with her. Because there was little or no time to train the staff who stayed with her, I continued to develop methods that were effective and easy to learn.

These methods seemed to be consistent and evolved into a one-sheet set of instructions that I entitled Ten Absolutes. Each chapter of this book is based on one of the "Ten Absolutes" as listed on the back cover. You may copy the Ten Absolutes as long as the copyright remains at the bottom. Keep them available for quick reference or give them to friends. If you find yourself on the NEVER side (and you will), don't despair just move over to the Right side and start again and your day will improve!

The most important thing of all is to understand that you need not feel guilty if you have been doing things "all wrong". What you need to do is understand that this is not an exact science and we are all human. There are no perfect people or perfect solutions to challenges. Use this book as a tool to assist you in enhancing quality of life for yourself and especially for the person with Alzheimer's Disease. It is my deepest and most sincere wish that this book will give you Help and Hope!

NEVER ARGUE

ALWAYS AGREE

Argue:
"You know your mother has been dead for years, you cannot wait for her to eat dinner."
Agree:
"I haven't seen your mother today, if I see her I will tell her you are looking for her, while we are waiting lets have a bite to eat."

NOW WHAT DOES THAT MEAN?

To never argue is probably a good idea for effective communication with everyone. Never arguing is essential when working with someone with Alzheimer's Disease.

The most common response to this suggestion, and you, the caregiver, believe this to be true, is that you really don't argue with the person with Alzheimer's Disease. Probably one of the more common sources of arguments is seen as "correcting" rather than "arguing". From your perspective, persons who are memory impaired are likely to make inaccurate statements or believe things that just aren't true. It becomes second nature to correct these inaccuracies and the justification for such corrections intends to help the confused person to be less confused.

However, if we believe the doctors have made an accurate diagnosis then we already know a person with Alzheimer's is not able to adequately or consistently process and learn new information. So, we need to learn and accept that they will not benefit from corrections. Actually, corrections are detrimental because the person with Alzheimer's becomes embarrassed, as they are aware that they have made a mistake. The bonus of avoiding corrections is that it will save face for them and eliminate the need to argue.

ARE THESE SCENARIOS FAMILIAR?

When you correct a person with Alzheimer's Disease they often respond in a manner that is very argumentative, will become upset, and often accuse you of things totally unrelated to the subject. The following are some examples that illustrate the point of agreeing instead of arguing. Hopefully you will see yourself in some of these scenarios and get a laugh out of them to realize that others have been down the same path and often.

Searching for someone who has died:

A very common occurrence, often the source of argument, unfortunately often labels the person as having delusions or hallucinations. An example of this is the incessant search for someone who is no longer alive. Often the search is for a parent and the person with Alzheimer's Disease might even refuse to eat because they are waiting for that parent. At this point most caregivers who have been encouraged "to agree" have problems with their ethic and value systems. They respond, "I can't agree with him or her. I have never lied to my spouse or parent before and I am not going to now". But the tool of agreeing is not to condone or encourage lying but it is to utilize kindness and understanding of the immediate needs for the person with Alzheimer's Disease. No one ever needs to relive the moment when they are told a loved one is dead. If the person with Alzheimer's Disease remembered that the person they are looking for is dead, then they wouldn't be looking for them. They are not asking you if that person is dead or alive, they are looking for them. It is likely that this person has been a source of comfort for them and they are in need of comfort, which is why they are searching. This person probably represents a substitution for a better place in time. It is honest and very kind to merely answer that you have not seen them today. If the person they are seeking is dead, you know you really haven't seen them today. It is even kinder to offer them reassurance, something that can never be overdone. This can be done in a variety of ways. The easiest and most effective seems to be for you to offer to tell the person with Alzheimer's Disease that if you see their loved one you will let them know. This will avoid an argument and downplay the event of looking for someone that no longer exists. It also offers you the opportunity to change the subject by introducing something that will fill their time, thus meeting their need and eliminating the search (for now).

Wanting to "go home":

The next most difficult and most often repeated phrase that is cause for serious argument is, "I want to go home." This phrase is so characteristic of the disease process it is the name of a chapter in the book written by Robinson, A, Spencer, B., & White, L. (1991). Understanding Difficult Behaviors. (2nd. Ed.). Ypsilanti, MI.:

Eastern Michigan University. It is usually very reassuring to discover that it is a common phenomenon. It is suggested that the search for home is once again a symbol for a search for a better place in time, something that offers comfort. It also has been suggested that it is a term for searching for their fading memory. Whatever the meaning behind the statement, it is not something that should create an argument. It is especially guilt provoking for the caregiver if the person has been in respite care or has recently moved into a 24-hr living alternative. When you see them, invariably they will say "I want to go home" and the immediate interpretation is they want to return to their most recent home. This automatically feeds into your anxiety about the recent change of events and creates questions, in your mind, about the decision. It is very easy to assume they are unhappy and they want to go home. This is a very common problem even for those who know that their loved one has always been asking to go home. Often, the only way to alleviate this concern, for you, is to actually take them home and then when they are there, you realize that they still continue to ask to go home. **Then you begin to understand that what they say is rarely what they mean.** It takes a great deal of practice and understanding on your part to tune into what they mean rather than what they say. When you become skilled at this interpretation, the frustration level for both of you will significantly decline and your quality of life will be improved.

What you should not do is tell them they are home. That statement creates the all time argument that often results in catastrophic reactions. What you need to do is tell them the truth and to do that you say, "SO DO I", then change the subject to another subject as quickly as possible. There are many ways to "go along" that are ethically truthful, validate their feelings, reassure them and best of all prevent arguments that needlessly frustrate and upset both of you.

We have covered the two most common sources for arguments and the most effective reactions are usually quite easy to adopt once they have been discussed. In addition, the idea that you don't argue with them has adequately been justified. You can rightfully say that persons with Alzheimer's Disease are very argumentative but you seldom see that what you personally say is arguing with them. It is time for you to think about a fact. It is impossible to argue with someone who does not argue; it usually takes two to argue. Now with this fact in mind, you will need to learn to not let them argue with you - which of course can simply be accomplished by your refusing to argue.

Not arguing and not correcting, this sounds easy until we get into the area of family dynamics. Another fact to remember, just because you have someone with Alzheimer's Disease in your family, all of the family dynamics, positive and negative, do not suddenly disappear. Actually, they begin to run rampant because all of you are stressed and feel GUILTY.

Untrue statements:

Let's assume that your 'favorite' sister comes to visit. She is the one who mom always liked best and consistent with your entire life story, the one who is too busy with her own life to help with mom. She only visits occasionally to comment on the things that seem to be wrong and to remind you that you need to have a life of your own! She comes in and immediately exclaims "Mother have you been losing weight?" to which your mother replies, " I haven't eaten in weeks". Now you really need to be able to defend yourself because your mother always eats and she just had lunch. So immediately you say, "Mother don't you remember we just had lunch and we had chips, ham and cheese croissants and your favorite fruit salad." Mom restates, " I haven't eaten in weeks". Your sister crosses her arms and says, "No wonder she is losing weight". You can argue and argue and everyone will become more and more upset and no one will remember lunch or you can simply say, "Well, then you must be hungry, why don't we have some coffee and cookies right now." You are agreeing and actually you are showing your sister that you will give her something to eat whenever she mentions food. You both do know that she can't remember when she last ate so don't make it an issue for anyone. This approach will benefit you and your mother because an argument is avoided.

Suppose you are the 'favorite' sister and you come to visit your father every day but your sister believes that she is the only one that ever visits. You say, "Hello, Dad how are you today?" and he says, "Where have you been, I haven't seen you in a long time?" Your immediate response is likely to be defensive. You will truthfully state you were there yesterday, to which he will truthfully not remember and repeat that he hasn't seen you for a long time. You can and will give him examples of what you did or talked about, which he will truly not remember and it goes on and on with both of you becoming unnecessarily upset. What you need to do instead is agree. You could say something like, "It is so wonderful to be missed, I will try to visit more often". Then give him a hug and go do some of the things he likes to do on your visits such as visit the ice cream parlor. It is likely that a staff person in the care facility will see you there, and know you by name, which is evidence of your visiting frequency. The payoff is that you are not upset and neither is your Dad. Arguing gets everyone upset and solves nothing because the person with Alzheimer's Disease truly can't remember. Not remembering is part of their disease.

It is no longer a secret that the theme of this book and the key to effective interactions is for YOU TO CHANGE. Changing and learning change will never become perfect, it will not work 100% of the time and at first it will be very difficult. This is true of everything we try in life. However, with practice and a little time you will find that the frustration level for both of you is significantly diminished.

It is acceptable for you to actually WHINE a bit while adjusting to the idea that you not only have had your entire life disrupted by this disease process and now YOU ARE THE ONE THAT HAS TO CHANGE - IT IS NOT FAIR!

YOU ARE ABSOLUTELY CORRECT IT IS NOT FAIR. This disease isn't fair and if it is fairness you are looking for, you are going to be very angry and disappointed. IF YOU ARE ANGRY AND DISAPPOINTED - GOOD FOR YOU!

You have a right to that anger and disappointment and you need to express that anger. It may be enough to express it and it can even be a way for siblings (family members) to agree on something. Often this can be an approach that will bring family members together. It is something you can do in response to this disease. With other diseases you can often help by making the ill person more comfortable. With the slow insidious nature of this disease and the feeling of hopelessness when trying to communicate, it is understandable that many people just "stay away". If there is a simple set of rules of communication and everyone is given the opportunity to see them work, then perhaps everyone can share some of the burden. For those who are close they can practice face to face, for those at a distance, they can practice by phone.

MOST IMPORTANT!

Probably the best way to describe the, "never argue-always agree" principle is to just go along with whatever they are saying and doing. It really can get to be a lot of fun for both of you if you can relax and enjoy the tone of the conversation. Take pleasure in interacting and just ignore the words.

NEVER REASON

ALWAYS DIVERT

<u>Reason:</u>
"You did not take a bath today and you need to take a bath because we have an appointment with the Doctor. Then we are going to go to lunch with Jane and then we are going to get you a new pair of shoes, and why are you walking off when I am talking to you. We have to go in here and get your bath and we have to hurry",

<u>Divert:</u>
" Please come in here with me. Oh, I know you aren't going to take a bath. Let me help with that shoe. Oh, I know you aren't going to take a bath. Just slide this off over your arm. Oh, I know you aren't going to take a bath. How does this water feel, it seems warm enough. Oh, I know you aren't going to take a bath. Just step right in here."

NOW WHAT DOES THAT MEAN?

As a society we talk in a manner that includes reasons for everything. No one is expected to do anything without a reason. Consequently we give lengthy reasons for everything we do with little or no thought. Because a person with Alzheimer's Disease usually has difficulty understanding, it is natural to assume that they need even more reasons. However, this is exactly the opposite of what they need. Even in the very early stages, their most recent memory is the most impaired which means they can not remember the most recent things you say. In addition, if they have problems with executive functioning, and many do, they have difficulty in planning anything. With reasoning we are expecting them to remember and plan - they cannot do this. It is the disease causing this and not a desire of the person with Alzheimer's Disease to be difficult.

With the best of intentions you are making it impossible for them to do what you want them to do. In addition, your reasoning is very frustrating as it comes across to them as incessant babbling in a manner that seems like a foreign language. Then when they don't respond, your babbling increases as you explain in more detail and the frustration you feel becomes evident in your body language. Your stress level shows in your body language and makes them frustrated and their response to your frustration is of embarrassment and hurt feelings. We now have entered that zone of no return - around and around and around - where will it end?

ARE THESE SCENARIOS FAMILIAR?
Preparation for an outing:

If the last time you and a person with Alzheimer's Disease went to the Doctor, or out for lunch, or shopping and the trip was a total disaster it does not mean that you will have to stop outings. What it means is that you need to do some things differently than you did last time. You need to see this as a new challenge and a new situation but you have new tools to use for practice. Don't plan too many things at once and don't talk about any of them. On a day that you have a lot to do YOU need to plan to keep the day structured as close to the normal routine as possible.

First things first, keep it simple and don't explain or try to get them to plan ahead. You need to plan ahead but not out loud and if the prospect of planning ahead stresses you out, then you need to find a way to do less. Concentrate on one task at a time, eating breakfast, and while the person with AD is still eating, get everything ready for the bath. If they are particularly slow, get yourself ready, except for your clothes, while you go back and forth offer encouragement, smiles and maybe even kisses. It is important to keep their daily routine, however, if bathing is problematic, it is very wise to skip the bathing on an outing day. There are ways to be clean without a complete bath and these ways need to be used and you need to be satisfied with the results. Actually, you need to learn to accept the results. Focus on what you are trying to accomplish and a successful outing is the object. If you start off with a bath you may both be too frustrated for the outing.

Bathing:

Don't make the bath a big deal but just a natural progression. Get them to walk with you to the bathroom, motion and touch, but don't talk. In the bathroom agree with them NEVER ARGUE, repeat what they say to you, then divert. "I know you already took a bath, feel how warm this water is. You aren't going to take a bath, let me help you get this shirt off. Put your foot right here, that is perfect. Hold this cloth, now rub here. Excellent! O.K. here is the towel, all done. You were a great help, thank you!" Focus on what you are doing, repeat what they say, divert to another subject and keep moving. The worst thing that can happen is that you might get wet - that is the reason you stay in your robe instead of getting dressed. If you don't live in the same home, you need to put something over your clothes so you don't get wet. The bath really is that simple if you don't REASON and you don't make it an issue and you don't ARGUE.

Dressing:

Now that the bath is over, they can get dressed. Do not let them choose their own clothing unless you will be happy with what they might choose. It is important that they have a choice in things but an outing day does not allow time for disagreement or the forum for creative dressing. Hand them the clothes you have already selected in the order to be put on. You can assist by anticipating their needs and saying very little. Good phrases are, "Try this, move your arm here, that is perfect, I wonder if this will work".

Doctor's Appointment:

Now that they are clean and dressed won't it be fun to go for a ride. Don't begin to explain where you are going. When you do address where you are going, answer with honest accurate succinct statements such as, "Downtown, in this parking garage, to the third floor, in this office". If they like going to the Doctor, then of course tell them you are going to the Doctor. You can continue to use the same techniques of repeating and diverting while you wait for the Doctor. "You are not going to see the Doctor? Do you want a piece of this candy? We will leave in a few minutes, look at this magazine article, I didn't know this. We will leave as soon as we can; do you want a piece of this candy?" Do not be embarrassed if they are not

28

cooperative with the Doctor, the Doctor needs to see the true picture. You need to stay calm and repeat what they say to the Doctor (which is often not accurate), such as, "Tom is feeling just fine but sometimes his head hurts". Keep it simple get the point across and DO NOT talk about them as if they are not there and your visit will be successful. Leaving will be the same process in reverse, stay calm and keep it simple. Don't offer too much information, one step at a time.

Eating out:

If all went well with the bath or doctor's appointment, then you can actually go to lunch. Go somewhere that requires no waiting time, is fairly quiet, and serves fast. If you are both tired be flexible, maybe have a friend get into your car, go through a drive-up window at a restaurant and eat at a picnic table in the park. Do what the person with Alzheimer's has always liked to do. If they never went out to lunch then prearrange to have them at home with a sitter (can be a friend or a relative) for lunch. Then you go to lunch with one of your friends, make time for yourself. Don't try to do shopping on the same day as a Doctor appointment and lunch. As you practice, you will have more successful outings and you can see when too much is too much. Getting it over with in one day can create a monster. When you are more successful with outings the prospect of another isn't so overwhelming - think of it as practice!

Preparation for visitors:

Your husband Tom, who has Alzheimer's Disease, and you are working around the house having a perfectly normal day. You say to Tom,

"Our good friends Jim and Alice are coming for dinner, why don't you go rest in your chair while I set the table. Really, I can do this, thank you for helping me but I can get this done because I still need to change my clothes - you just go and relax for a few minutes. No, please don't take that silverware to the kitchen I am trying to set the table. Tom, I can do this myself, please go watch television for awhile, please let me take care of this. Oh, never mind do whatever you want. That is what you are going to do anyway - I am going to go and change my clothes! Now why are you following me in here, I just need to change my clothes and I will be out, we need to hurry so we are ready when our guests get here."

When friends are coming over, you might want your loved one to get rest before they arrive. You may need to go with the person with Alzheimer's Disease to his chair and get him settled. It will take more time in the beginning but will be worth the time. Keep down the anticipation and maybe not even tell him until the guests are coming up the walk. He may not process that someone is coming but he will process the feeling of anticipation and the anticipation will make it impossible for him to rest. If he can't settle into his chair then give him something else he truly likes to do, even if it makes a mess, to keep him busy and content. Keeping him occupied will keep your frustration level down and therefore, he won't sense and adopt the same level of frustration. Telling yourself not to be frustrated is not going to work for you; you need to do something to change the situation if you are getting frazzled. Don't feel guilty and frustrated with yourself if you lose your cool; in the years of your relationship you have lost your cool before and sometimes it helped - do not think that a relationship should be perfect because your spouse has Alzheimer's. No relationship is ever perfect or without conflict - don't expect the impossible.

MOST IMPORTANT!

You have a goal in mind and you probably have too many things to do especially if your activities involve the person with Alzheimer's. Whether it is going about the routine of the day that includes that troublesome bath, an outing for fun, appointments, or guests coming for dinner the focus must shift from reasoning with them to what needs to be accomplished. This is what I laughingly refer to as a TMI (Too Much Information) issue. They cannot process all of this information and they need to be calm and comfortable for the events to be successful. They cannot be calm and comfortable unless you remain calm and comfortable. So, we are back to YOU.

Don't give up outings because they are too difficult. Find ways to make them less difficult yet more enjoyable for both of you. It is important to maintain what have always been your favorite outings even if you have to change the structure and reduce the time spent.

Focus on the task to be done and concentrate only on one task at a time. Divert their attention from the thing that is getting them stuck. Divert their attention from negative behaviors. Diversion always works if you can divert to their favorite foods and activities and you must know what those favorite things are. Anyone that helps in providing care must also know his or her favorite things.

Go along with them but do what needs to be done. They rarely say what they mean and they don't understand and keep track of everything you say. They do seem to have an uncanny knack of picking up the one or two words that you didn't want them to process and then they focus on just those words. This is the reason for the diversion and why it is successful. If you agree with them with your response, not necessarily in content, and then divert to the task at hand or their favorite things you can accomplish a lot in a short period of time. They cannot respond positively to being rushed! They will respond negatively to your frustration because they cannot hurry.

NEVER SHAME

ALWAYS DISTRACT

Shame:
   "How can you accuse John of stealing your things after all he has done for us?"
Distract:
   "John is here to help us find your wallet, lets have a cup of coffee and get started."

NOW WHAT DOES THAT MEAN?

Probably one of the greatest misconceptions about Alzheimer's Disease is that the person who has the disease has impaired feelings. This is not true. They do have memory impairment that results in cognitive problems. Cognition pertains to the mental process of perception, memory, judgment and reasoning. It doesn't mean feelings. THEIR FEELINGS ARE INTACT, THEIR FEELINGS ARE NOT IMPAIRED.

If you have thought about this at any time, you are already very aware of the heightened awareness and increased sensitivities of a person with Alzheimer's Disease. You will probably find that they are more sensitive and probably show more affection than they have in their entire life. They seem to sense things and react to things like they have never done before.

It is probably true that most everyone understands that when you are talking about feelings in relation to the heart, the reference is not about the organ in the left side of our chest that pumps the blood through our body. We are really

33

referring to the section of our brain that controls feelings and emotions. It is important to establish that most people separate these subjects we think of as feelings, as coming from the heart not the head. The often heard statement "Intellectually I understand, but I am still having difficulty accepting it. I just feel like there is something else.", is evidence of a separation, in our minds eye, of intellect versus feelings. The reference to "gut" and "intuition" even though vague seems to indicate that we can feel something even if we can't back it up with evidence, statistics, or proof. The entire right brain-left brain phenomenon of the 1980's seemed to be based on feelings versus intellect. The point of presenting this information is to emphasize the knowledge that cognition and feelings are different, and they are different for everyone. IT IS ESSENTIAL THAT YOU UNDERSTAND AND ACCEPT THAT A PERSON WITH ALZHEIMER'S DISEASE IS COGNITIVELY IMPAIRED NOT FEELING IMPAIRED.

In the mid-1980's I had the opportunity to attend a Nancy Mace workshop. She started her lecture by requesting a show of hands of those persons who remembered the name of the mathematics class they took in eighth grade. She then asked for a show of hands of those who remembered their first love. As one might suspect there were no hands raised for the first question but all hands raised for the second. For a decade I asked that same question at my presentations. Through the years there have been a few persons that raised their hand to the first question. For those who were over 25 years old there was general agreement that they remembered the class because they were either particularly good or particularly poor at math. No one remembered enough about their mathematics class to put a problem from that class on the board and explain it to the audience.

The point of this exercise was to show that intellectual things, like mathematics, don't last very long or aren't important through the years. Where as feelings and emotions on the other hand remain in our memories for a lifetime.

There is an old wives tale that states if you lose your sight you can hear better. It seems that for the person with Alzheimer's Disease, as their ability to express and understand thoughts decline, their feelings intensify.

Embarrassment for example is clearly a strong feeling which is often visible with the flushing of the skin as one turns red. If all feelings are heightened rather than impaired then it is understandable that a person with Alzheimer's is easily embarrassed. It is very kind and incredibly important as a friend, loved one, caregiver and protector to assist the person with Alzheimer's Disease in avoiding embarrassment.

Unfortunately, the embarrassment is easy to misinterpret. The natural inclination for the caregiver seems to be to avoid ones own embarrassment about what the person with Alzheimer's does. This seems to be done, with the best of intentions, by pointing out their errors and correcting them. It will be much less embarrassing for them and probably will go unnoticed if you can learn to discreetly ignore errors and quickly distract to a better subject or activity. The only risk in this is that it might appear that you are oblivious to a problem. If you rethink many situations, being oblivious should be preferable to becoming the center of attention when a situation escalates or totally "gets out of hand".

ARE THESE SCENARIOS FAMILIAR?
Accusations of Theft:

Accusations of theft are often a source of embarrassment for both the person with Alzheimer's Disease and their primary caregiver. The person with Alzheimer's Disease is often labeled as paranoid and will accuse family, friends and strangers of theft of their misplaced items. It is important to learn a proactive approach to accusations of theft. Usually, the accused is aware that the person with AD has received a diagnosis or at least is having some significant problems in the areas of behavior. The family or friends probably don't really need an apology and if they do, it can be done at a better time. The explanation or apology should definitely not be done in front of the person with Alzheimer's Disease, as it will be very embarrassing and we always need to try to avoid embarrassing them. Ignore the accusation. Discuss the issue. For example if a friend and neighbor, John stops by and the person with AD has just angrily said, "Don't let him in here he stole my wallet." Your response, to avoid embarrassment could be, "John, it is so nice of you to stop by. Tom is missing his wallet and we thought you might assist in finding it since you help so often. Before we begin the search why don't we have a cup of coffee." Focus on the diversion, coffee, get to a happier subject and try to enjoy the visit.

If your friend John really doesn't understand, then a later discreet telephone call can provide explanations, but do not explain in front of the person with Alzheimer's Disease. Initially, this may be a very important telephone call as it can provide you with someone to talk to about your loved one's condition. It also could be a wonderful way to teach them how to work effectively with your loved one and this also sets up a network for assistance for you. Turn a negative into a positive and begin to build a support system for you and for the person with Alzheimer's Disease.

Do You Remember Me?

What to say when someone comes up and says, "Do you remember me?", to which they say no or don't reply at all? Instead of saying, "Of course you remember Alice." You could say, "Alice, you are certainly looking younger every day, I almost didn't recognize you. We are late for an appointment right now but I will call soon."

It seems important to digress just a moment here to try to understand why well intentioned friends and family members insist on asking a memory impaired person if they remember. No one would ever consider asking a person that had just gone blind if they have read any good books lately. It appears that the reason memory impaired persons are questioned is because the persons most concerned about them want to disprove they are memory impaired. If anyone asks the person with AD questions and the answers are right then the diagnosis is a mistake, the problem will go away and 'everyone can live happily ever after.' The psychological term for this hopeful belief system is called denial. It is important to understand this denial in ourselves and everyone else and then we can deal with the issue in a way that is not defensive and prevents embarrassment for the person with Alzheimer's Disease.

It is helpful to prompt a person with Alzheimer's Disease when you approach them. Be aware that it has to become unimportant to you if they can't remember you by name. Always offer your name, not so they remember it, they are unlikely to be able to store that new information but so they are put at ease and can concentrate on positive interactions not 'saying the correct thing.' For example you can say "Hi, Mom, it is Sarah," not "Hi, Mom do you know me today". If you are approaching a friend who you have heard has Alzheimer's Disease say "Hi, Tom it is your counterpart from General Electric, it is so good to see you." Then talk in general terms, make small talk, the weather, and life in general, etc. Just visit for the pleasure of interacting. Don't spend your time on diagnostic investigation. Wouldn't you just hate to think that everyone you spoke to for the rest of your life was analyzing your words to see how much you knew today? That kind of pressure would make a memory wizard anxious, and imagine what it must do to someone who is literally suffering with the ravages of memory loss.

Theft? When they take things that belong to someone else:

If a person with AD "helps themselves" to

things such as taking a drink of something at the table that belongs to someone else, just call for the waiter and order a replacement with no explanation. If it happens in a home, just say something to the hostess like, "I need to get a new glass for this drink, may I help myself in the kitchen?" If it happens because you have stopped by a table on your way out of the restaurant, just place a dollar on the table and be on your way, sincerely ask the person with whom you have stopped to visit to call you. Take ownership of the problem by solving it in the least conspicuous way possible and so it appears that something natural happened. Do not draw attention to the situation in any way and DO NOT address the person with AD about the situation it is very embarrassing for them. The most common response to embarrassment, for a person with Alzheimer's Disease is to become defensive and then they actually will forget why they are defensive. They will remain defensive and you now have "gotten the bad feelings going, the good feelings are lost and a truly embarrassing situation can erupt for everyone involved".

It is a prudent practice to generally avoid stopping by tables in restaurants, standing in corridors talking, etc. it can be boring and confusing and is a place for creating many awkward situations. Smile, wave and move on as if you are late for an appointment. If it is someone you want to visit with or have been meaning to call, this can be a wonderful opportunity for you to later make a phone call or write a note. You can start out with an apology for not having time to visit the other day and if it is appropriate can share the information about the disease. In the initial conversation of informing someone that the person you were with has Alzheimer's Disease, the person receiving the news will almost always ask what he or she can do. This is the opportunity for caregivers to practice two things: 1. explain the disease in a positive light and 2. open the avenue for asking these friends for assistance with this journey. This will be discussed more in the last chapter of this book.

Inappropriate language/disparaging remarks:
Many caregivers state that their mother, spouse etc. would never have used profanity and now they 'sound like a sailor'. This usually makes me smile because it seems that we are now able to hear what they were really thinking all along but, these people had been taught 'especially as proper young ladies' that they couldn't use foul language. If you, as caregivers, can get over the shock of the unexpected or improper curse words, this is a situation that can truly hold some humor. Humor is in short supply for a caregiver and there are a lot of studies that say 'humor is good medicine.' Try to see some humor in this pristine little lady spewing profanity at some person that has just embarrassed her and or insulted her intelligence. Practice not being shocked, make statements like, "Well I guess we got that settled", rather than appearing shocked or outraged or even insulted. On the flip side, you also need to control your humor so that you in no way appear to be laughing at the person with Alzheimer's Disease. Once again it isn't really the words that you use, it is your tone or attitude that is

coming through not just to the person with AD but to you as well.

Sometimes they make a disparaging (though often honest) remark about size, clothing, deformity, color etc. Do not address the remark, but ignore it and quickly and efficiently change the subject by saying something like this, "The chocolate store we are looking for is over this way." You cannot apologize in front of the person with Alzheimer's Disease, because they will deny having said anything. The person with AD can not learn to keep their remarks to themselves. The person insulted, if they even heard, will be more insulted if the conversation continues. Distract to a better subject quickly!

Incontinence:

Incontinence can be a very embarrassing and frustrating issue for both the person with Alzheimer's Disease and their caregivers. This is especially difficult if it is in public and they are visibly wet or soiled which results in soiling car seats and upholstery. First, and most importantly this needs to be avoided, by having them go to the toilet regularly and by knowing or learning their toileting patterns. If this doesn't prevent the problem and they are truly having accidents they should wear a disposable undergarment. There is a relatively new product (pull-ups) now that is comfortable, hardly shows, is totally disposable, and holds a great deal of liquid. It is an essential tool for managing incontinence without unnecessary embarrassment. However, for those times when wetness is apparent, it is always a good plan to carry a small bag with at least a sweater in it. Say to them, "You must be cold". Tie the sweater around their waist, with the largest part covering either front or back as most needed and then get to a place to change clothing. Never point out the fact that they are wet. Get them to go with you under "false pretenses" if you must, but do not state the obvious. In most cases, they already know and it is already embarrassing to them.

Cleaning up someone who has been incontinent is also very embarrassing for them and they may not want you to assist. Obviously, you need to assist but this needs to be handled very delicately and it may take a little time. It is always better to try to solve this problem in a familiar place and you are aware that in a public restroom it will be more difficult. It will become very important for you to plan ahead and know your territory and then you can have successful outings even with a person who is incontinent, but you need to be prepared. Take supplies, at least a sweater to carry with you for immediate cover up. Frequent places with family and or handicapped restrooms where you can comfortably go into the restroom with them even if they are members of the opposite sex. Disposable wipes and a disposable undergarment can actually fit in a small take along bag that they can carry in the form of a fanny pack. Have some disposable cover-up pads under the front seat or in the trunk of the car so you can cover and protect the seat if you need to make a hasty trip home. Most of all don't get overly flustered, don't embarrass the person who just had an accident and plan better for the next time if things didn't work out this time.

MOST IMPORTANT!

This subject of embarrassment and unnecessarily shaming comes up much more often than you realize. Please become aware of it, as it is often the cause of many unnecessary "flare-ups" and tends to be the kind of thing that creates "bad feelings". Once those "bad feelings" get started they tend to snowball. This is true for everyone, not just for a person with Alzheimer's Disease. You know how quickly your good mood changes to a bad one when someone insults you or hurts your feelings! Think about it, how long does it take and what does it take to get you back in a good mood?

The person with AD may not be able to remember what hurt their feelings but the feelings stay with them, build, and come out later at a very unexplainable and inappropriate time. Thus the explanation of, " The person with AD for no reason just became very angry, blew up, pushed her, shook his fist, etc.", is probably not accurate. There could have been many reasons "bad feelings" had built through the day. Unfortunately, these reasons just aren't apparent at the time of the reaction to them.

Keep "good feelings" going as much as possible. Avoid " bad feelings" that means ignore errors and inappropriate behaviors, usually by distracting to some favorite things. If the first attempt is not successful and they become more upset then APOLOGIZE, even if you have not done anything wrong. BE SINCERE, NEVER SARCASTIC, you can always honestly be sorry about the situation. Apologizing will be an advantage to both of you. Say, "I am so sorry that happened, but nothing less than a nice long walk, cup of tea, chocolate bar, etc. will make it better." Then take that walk, get that tea or chocolate bar. Depending on their level of interaction, don't be too quick. You may need to commiserate a few minutes with statement like, "Don't you just hate when that happens, when it happens to me I just want to cry, scream, kick the wall, etc. but then it just gets worse and worse (shake your head, frown). We might feel better if we take a long walk, have a cup of tea, eat a chocolate bar, etc."

KEEP THOSE GOOD FEELINGS GOING YOU BOTH REALLY NEED THEM! This brings to mind an old song that I loved as a child and used to sing with my Grandma. The words as I remember them were, "Accentuate the positive, eliminate the negative, don't mess with Mr. in-between". This would be an excellent theme song for avoiding embarrassment and negative discourse in providing care for a person with Alzheimer's Disease!

NEVER LECTURE

ALWAYS REASSURE

Lecture:
"You have got to go back to bed and get some sleep.
You have been up half the night and why on earth did
you empty these drawers? Who is supposed to clean
up this mess? I suppose tomorrow you will want to
sleep all day and we won't be able to go to Carol's
house and help with the children. I am just too tired to
deal with this so you have to get in bed and go to sleep
right now. We can't continue like this, no one can live
this way, we both have got to get some sleep."
Reassure:
"I can't sleep either. Let's go to the bathroom. I
need something to drink (give them a drink). Try to lie
down again (pat the bed). No? How about some
cookies and milk. Try to lie down again (sit beside the
bed & pat the bed). Doesn't that feel good." (Stay
until settled or asleep, rub their hand, forehead, arm).

NOW WHAT DOES THAT MEAN?

One of the most acknowledged books about
this disease The 36-Hour Day, Nancy L. Mace &
Peter V. Rabins, M.D. (1981, 84) Warner Books,
New York, N.Y., is accurately depicted with the
title. This is true, you will live a 36 Hour Day,
especially if you have communication problems
with the Alzheimer's person and specifically if you
are trying to care for them without assistance.

There are two things that are essential to get
through the progression of this disease and
maintain any quality of life for both you and the
person with Alzheimer's Disease. First, you must

learn to understand the disease so you can change how you approach the secondary symptoms and second, you must be willing to ask for and accept assistance. This is not easy but is also not optional. The statistics on what happens to the primary caregiver of a person with Alzheimer's Disease are truly frightening. The person with Alzheimer's Disease truly needs you to be there to care and advocate for them. If you do not find a way to do this from the beginning, they are likely to outlive you and then it is questionable as to what will happen to them. This is not just for spouses it applies to children and siblings as well. Do not allow the stress of caring for someone with this disease destroy you. If they can not manage without you for an hour, a day, a week, a month what will they do for a lifetime?

The example at the beginning of the chapter is a very familiar scenario of everyday life dialog between a person with Alzheimer's Disease and their primary caregiver. The frustration is exhibited with lengthy lectures that often include everything from pleas to threats.

Lecturing doesn't work. It may possibly be an outlet for your stress and frustration but it is dangerous and counterproductive. A person with AD can become very angry which could possibly result in physical confrontations. Most certainly, you will always feel guilty after you have interacted in this manner. What you need to do instead is provide reassurance. The reassurance will help you as well as them and it is truly not that difficult to change from lecturing to reassurance. It will take practice and you can't practice unless you try.

ARE THESE SCENARIOS FAMILIAR?

Look at the example at the beginning of the chapter. The person with AD has been up all night wandering around and rummaging through drawers. You are in a state of sheer exhaustion. You have been able to sleep only long enough for him/her to have spent time rummaging and rearranging closets and chest of drawers. You really just want to go back to sleep but both of you will be totally frustrated and unable to sleep if you have angry exchanges. Instead of lecturing, you can state the facts but in a different way.

"Don't you want to go back to bed and sleep? You must be tired. It looks like you have worked all night, tomorrow we can do some serious drawer rearranging. We need to get a little snack. How about cookies and milk. Isn't this good? I am so glad we thought of it. Now, if you will lie down I will rub your shoulders a bit and you can go off to "slumberland". We have a wonderful day planned tomorrow and you don't want to be sleepy."

The talk is positive and reassuring though honest, you probably can laugh if you think of the messed up drawers as a project. Going to the bathroom, getting something to eat and to drink is a natural way to create a scenario for sleep (for you too). Rubbing forehead, arms, back etc. are very soothing and will often relax the person with AD enough that they go to sleep. Then because you aren't angry or guilty and you are exhausted you too will go right back to sleep. If it doesn't work the first time try the cycle again, toilet, something to drink, something to eat and massage to get back to sleep.

MOST IMPORTANT!

Whenever they do something that doesn't make any sense to you and makes a lot of work for you it is very reasonable for you to be upset. However, this is when you need to blame the disease process. Accept and understand that they are not doing it because they want you to be miserable. Acceptance takes practice and will not happen immediately. It will take time for you to get to the place when you understand it is their disease and you will learn to react without anger. It might help to think about other diseases and their resultant messy, work producing attributes. You know that no one ever vomits, bleeds, has diarrhea or seizures just so they can create a mess for someone to clean up; they do it because it happens as a part of their condition. It is not controllable. However, for example, once you know someone has the flu, or a bleeding disorder, or a seizure disorder you can prepare for the symptoms. Being prepared results in less work. You can prepare for dealing with a person with AD and thereby, you can eliminate a lot of the frustration. This will make it much easier for you to be accepting and creative if you see it as a disease process.

Yes, you can prepare for this disease process. Many of the persons with AD need a safe area where they can move stuff around and it won't make any difference. If they are up a lot at night, then change their room to a creative safe place at night. Move the stuff out of their drawers that are important and leave items that don't matter; add items they seem to be the most drawn to and fill those drawers with these items. Moving, sorting, folding, packing are all safe activities and can be done with little or no attention from a caregiver. Get some nice boxes, perhaps a suitcase or two and encourage them to rummage and pack. You can converse about these items when you wake up and check on them but be kind. Don't ask or try to figure out what they are doing because it won't make sense to you, and they don't know. However, in their mind, they may be thinking of or planning for a trip. They will often mention the trip so discuss trips, maybe even some that you have taken. Listen, say words that may trigger old memories. Don't be curious or perplexed by what they are doing; they are keeping busy and they are obviously content - enjoy don't disturb those moments. When the stuff gets soiled, if washable, sort it by color, run it through the washer and dryer and return it when clean. They will fold, unfold sort etc. If it isn't washable you might need to discard and replace with like items. Get some things at the thrift store if you need extra stuff. If initial disorganization makes them uncomfortable put it all back in the drawers but be aware that they will take it out again. If they like to put on many outfits at the same time, fill the closets and drawers with clothing a bit too large for them so it is easier to take the clothes off again. If they like mail and paperwork give them a desk or card table and some boxes or bags of mail. Let them sort and look at those old boxes of receipts, greeting cards etc. that are in the attic. It might be interesting enough for you to rummage through things with them. Do not use valuables as they often tear and shred things. If they used a briefcase get several. Ladies like purses with many zippers and pockets, maybe a drawer of things that belong in purses (remember safety - avoid everything not edible or small enough to cause airway problems if swallowed.). Make it easy for yourself and keep them occupied. Tailor things to be as adult and as much in their lifelong interest areas as possible; pay attention to what they are doing and expand on it. Stop looking at it as crazy and stop trying to understand it. Use it to your advantage and in the long run to theirs. They are much better off rummaging around in a room than trying to get out the front door or following you around asking repetitive questions because they are bored.

Sometimes the mechanics of this really seem to be difficult for the caregivers, and it seems to be most difficult for spouses and siblings who live in the same home. With any other illness it doesn't seem unusual to even bring a hospital bed into the living room to accommodate "staying at home". There is often even Medicare money available to add ramps, rebuild doors and bathrooms, and lower countertops when an illness handicaps someone. Homes are always adjusted as the family situation changes, guestrooms become nurseries, cribs move out for bigger beds, furniture goes to college and comes back. With this disease process it seems like "Custer's Last Stand" to be willing to give them a room, dresser, closet etc. where they can rummage. Perhaps the adjustment can be made easier for you if you can view it as modifying the home for their disease.

Yes, once again it is the primary caregiver asked to change. This big change is likely to require you to give up the guestroom or even your room and you moving to the guest room. This big change could serve a personal purpose for you. Maybe it is a good time to sort out old things that you don't need and empty a closet. Make a small investment in underbed storage or install a closet organizer.

This is probably a good place to address the feeling of guilt that comes from the resentment of this disease, which has not only changed your life but it has also started changing your environment. It is perfectly normal to feel anger and to be angry at the disease. You need to focus the anger on the disease not on the behaviors of the person who is afflicted with the disease. As you well know it isn't easy for them either. If you can both pull together and do something to fight against the disease and also in the meantime, accommodate the person with the disease then you can express your feelings, grow and enjoy your loved one just as they are!

Keeping this in mind you really need to be aware of how much change is required to accept and live with this disease. Change is difficult for everyone even if it is positive change and it will be stressful. With this disease process, change and stress don't discriminate they both effect everyone. It is stressful for friends, spouses, siblings, parents, children and grandchildren. It is very unfair and you have a right and a need to express this anger. It is unlikely that you are going to be able to work through this anger and change without some assistance. Support groups are a wonderful resource where you can share some of these concerns. Even if you are one of those people who never ask for or need help, eventually the stress will even get to you! This disease is further complicated as it can last for years; the average is 8 years. It is nearly impossible to go through this journey with a loved one for years and not feel the adverse impact. I will say it again, you cannot handle this alone and you should not try, you must ask for assistance and then be willing to accept the assistance.

NEVER ASK THEM TO REMEMBER

LEARN TO REMINISCE

Remember:
"Do you remember who this is? What did you have for lunch today? Did Mary visit today? "When did Jeanne come to visit?"
Reminisce:
"Hi, Tom this is Sarah visiting with me from Elmhurst Elementary PTA. I had the nicest lunch today. Mary is such a pleasant person and she visits often. I hoped I would get here before Jeanne's visit."

NOW WHAT DOES THAT MEAN?

This is the area where everyone makes the most mistakes and please don't feel guilty. You really didn't know it was incorrect, just **change this right away**. In order for a person to have a diagnosis of Dementia of the Alzheimer's or any other type of dementia, a person has to have memory impairment (impaired ability to learn new information or to recall previously learned information) to the extent that it affects their everyday life. If they have this diagnosis then they can't remember, so wouldn't it be incredibly unkind to repeatedly ask them if they remember things?

As referred to in chapter 3, the never shame or embarrass section, you wouldn't ask a person who had just gone blind if they had read any good books lately. Would you ask a leg amputee to go for a walk? Why do we ask a person with memory impairment if they remember? I am not suggesting that it is done to be unkind, however, I am suggesting that it is indeed unkind. It appears that we do it usually because that is the way we all converse - we are socialized to ask information as a means of communicating.

It appears that often we ask them to remember mainly to see if maybe they are getting their memory back. The 1990's buzzword for that is DENIAL and it is a very real part of the grief process you are experiencing as you are dealing with what this disease process does to someone you love. It takes the person, on an intellectual level, that you have known and loved, and turns them into someone you may not recognize. It is perfectly understandable that you just want to keep checking, keep hoping that it is all a mistake, and it will go away. When the person with AD has the right answer to the question, and they sometimes do, (though you don't know whether to believe them as they also make up answers) then there is that glimmer of hope that they are misdiagnosed. Perhaps understanding why you might continue to ask them to remember will allow you to change this habit.

Reminiscing is different than remembering and reminiscing is one of the things that you can do very effectively. The brain degeneration of Alzheimer's disease is often referred to as regressive. In very lay terms this means that they lose information in reverse order that it was stored. Consequently, the things from today and yesterday are likely to not be stored at all but things from twenty years ago may be as clear as if they took place yesterday. This is why reminiscing about the past is so important and can provide you with hours of successful and enjoyable communication.

Like everything else, reminiscing can be much more effective if you learn a few skills. Asking direct questions about anything is something that needs to be avoided. This is not really just for an Alzheimer's person, don't you just hate it when people ask you direct questions? Often, you may not know the answer or you may just not think it is any of their business and there just isn't a nice way to impart that information. In the case of a person with Alzheimer's Disease it is even more complicated. They may not really comprehend the question; or they may fear that they will give the wrong answer so it is easier to become defensive, or just walk off.

Now that we have established that direct questions are not appropriate then it would appear that reminiscing is not possible. However, it is very possible and also very effective. The way to make reminiscing work is to let them tell you where they are and be the one with the information. Don't you just love to be called on when you do know the answer and isn't it fun to be the one that knows the most about a subject. Imagine how wonderful it would be if you had Alzheimer's Disease and you had the information and it was accurate. This is why reminiscing is so successful, because they often can remember the past. The technique for reminiscing is to allow them to tell everything their own way. The prompting needs to be with you not knowing the answers. For example: when looking at a photo album say, "That looks like Tom," they will quickly look at the picture and say that isn't Tom that is Jack and he is standing in front of the family home on Chestnut Street. Once they are comfortable they can go on and on with little or no prompting. The most common problem they get into while sharing information is interruptions. If they get interrupted they usually just need to start again. The same procedure can be used again by saying, "Could that possibly be Aunt Ellen when she was a teenager". It doesn't really make a lot of difference if they remember things accurately and correcting them will not be beneficial. It is O.K. to say that you thought otherwise but then dismiss it as if you were wrong. If you weren't a part of their life at that time, you won't even know if the information is accurate. What does matter is that you are enjoying yourselves and you are communicating and that keeps those good feelings going.

A bonus in reminiscing is that it will give you a clue as to how much they do remember and at what place in time they seem to be in their memory. This information can give you a great deal of insight to things they are searching for or talking about. If they are primarily in the 1940's then it is no wonder they think they aren't at home even if you have lived in your present home for 30 years. This is information you accumulate through reminiscing but not by asking direct questions.

During reminiscing often curiosity takes over and the temptation is great to ask a lot of questions to verify what you are thinking. It will not take you long to realize that pleasant effective reminiscing can come to an abrupt end if it becomes a question and answer session.

ARE THESE SCENARIOS FAMILIAR?

Questioning can be frustrating for everyone. A person with AD is rarely if ever able to remember what they had for lunch and actually whether they ate at all, to them, is a mystery. This is why they will say they haven't eaten for days or they will list a menu of something that doesn't even resemble what they actually had to eat. They might actually be recalling a meal they had fourteen years ago.

They can't remember accurately, if at all, but sometimes the thing that is remembered often provides just little enough information for you both to be even more frustrated. Questioning them is not only inappropriate, but it doesn't provide reliable information, so don't question!

MOST IMPORTANT!

Do not expect the family to be drawn closer through this process of stress and dealing with this disease. As you know, caregiving can be very stressful. You need to determine what you need for yourself and what is needed for the person with the Disease. Then a plan needs to be made to determine how care will be acquired.

Usually the responsibility of caring for a person with Alzheimer's Disease is not evenly distributed. Family dynamics are unlikely to improve at a time like this and often the person with Alzheimer's Disease is the one in the middle of a lot of unspoken conflict. Consequently, the frequency of someone's visits, their level of interaction, and the perception of involvement is often questioned and obviously inappropriately determined by questioning the person with Alzheimer's Disease.

It is very common and certainly a point of increased stress when it appears that the only assistance family members have to offer is criticism, especially those who are out of town or out of touch with the real situation. Do not let yourself get caught up in this, as personally as it is directed, you need to refuse to take responsibility for their expression of insecurity and guilt. Do not become defensive, but explain what you are doing and why. Be very matter of fact and provide them with information of what they can do to make things better. This may seem uncomfortable at first but it is important that you not share the total responsibility of a family member with AD. It will take practice for you to let go and to ask for help, but do not ask them for assistance - assume that they will provide assistance. They have the same genetic relationship with the person with AD as you do. You will also have to let go and offer appreciation not criticism if they do things in a way differently than you would. Very often family issues are about lifelong dynamics and about control. However, this is not a journey that works well alone and you need to step past those things and concentrate on the needs of the person with Alzheimer's Disease. The person with AD needs for you to take care of yourself and to not carry this burden all alone or they will not have you and that is the worst thing that can happen to them.

Having the person with AD attend a senior center or Alzheimer's Day Center will give you time for yourself but more importantly it will provide them with friends and a purpose in their daily life. If a day/care facility is available in your area then you should take advantage of the service. If there are funds for this option then they should be used and without guilt. If what is needed has an expense attached then it is simple to offer family members choices. A note to the family members to help in assuming their responsibilities is not out of line and is often effective. It can read or go something like this: "Mother is doing quite well but we have reached a point where she needs outside stimulation. The cost is $30 a day, payable in advance. Please mail your share of the cost ($150) directly to (divide the total bill for each sibling not including yourself) give the address. In the future you will receive a monthly bill."

If you need a weekend a month off then that too needs to be arranged. This can be done with a family member coming to the home where the person with Alzheimer's Disease lives - this is usually the least disruptive. Alternatives might be for them to spend a weekend with a family member or at a place that provides respite care. If these options are unavailable then you might need to hire a person to come to the house to stay with them. If funds are not available for these options then the same assumption of dividing the cost, can be made with family members.

If there really is no family then there must be close friends. It is not only O.K. to ask friends for assistance, in a situation such as this, it is necessary. Even if assistance is not monetary it can be supportive and a way to get a break. People really do often want to help but they usually just don't know what to do. The Alzheimer's Association now has a wonderful pamphlet available that gives 10 suggestions of how to assist the family of a person with Alzheimer's Disease. Pick up some of these and have them available to give to people who offer to help or who remind you to take care of yourself.

The Alzheimer's Association is also an excellent source for resources.

NEVER SAY, "I TOLD YOU"

ALWAYS REPEAT & REGROUP

I Told You:
"I just told you that we are not going to the bank today, it is Sunday and the bank is closed, how many times do I have to tell you we are not going to the bank it is Sunday"

Repeat, Regroup:
"Wouldn't you know it is too late for Church and we have to go to the bank tomorrow. Since it is Sunday, let's have Fried Chicken. Yes, we will go to the bank when it opens tomorrow."

NOW WHAT DOES THAT MEAN?

Repetitive behavior is not present in all persons with Alzheimer's Disease. Even those that don't have seriously repetitive behavior can sometimes become focused on one subject and thus will repeat it until they will truly drive you to distraction. This is when a sense of humor is essential and the ability to laugh at oneself a key for survival. In addition, it is often a sign that they truly are bored and need something to do.

The most obvious solution is to find them something to do that they will enjoy and can (repetitively) stick with for awhile. That is often a lot easier said than done, so these tips are for when attempts to keep them occupied doesn't work, though we will ultimately get back to that as the long term solution.

Repeating things over and over are just a part of what must be done. It is important to try to keep the answer the same and often writing it down, for them, will provide the assurance they need and the relief you need.

When they persist, you can repeat and repeat until you actually feel yourself escalating (talking louder, gritting your teeth) and then it is as with every behavior-time to try distraction. Always distract to favorite things and activities. Now my assumption is that you have already done this with them initially and repeatedly and it is just not working. The distraction I am actually suggesting now is for YOU and that is called regrouping. You may literally need to go out of the room or house and come back in again.

This is literal in meaning. Go out of the room and come back. Excuse yourself, go to the bathroom and shut the door wait a few minutes, and then come back. This will not necessarily change the subject but it will change your state of mind and that is usually what is needed to effectively change the subject.

I often share my story of this situation when I just couldn't take the repetition one more second. I knew it wasn't her fault but it wasn't my fault either and I just couldn't answer again. I went to the bathroom and closed the door and of course she followed me and was knocking. I didn't want to scare her but I just couldn't go back out so I flushed the toilet, turned on the water grabbed a towel and wrapped it around my head and screamed. The moment I did that I began to laugh which was what I needed. They do call that primal scream therapy and it was obviously extreme, but it worked. After that I would just think about it and would occasionally say to her that I was going to the bathroom to scream. Just visualizing myself in the bathroom screaming was all it took to realize that it wasn't really all that bad. What I needed was simply to stop what we were doing and take a few minutes to enjoy each other.

Going out and coming back in again is symbolic for taking time to do something that is enjoyable, taking a break. Have a cup of coffee or tea, go for a walk, call someone on the phone, play a favorite song and dance. It will break the repetition and it will prevent the need to scream or cry or both. It works and it is simple and you will get the most benefit.

Now how can you do that when you are so frustrated you could scream? Well it isn't easy and that is why you need to have a sense of humor and be able to laugh at yourself. Literally GO OUT AND COME BACK IN AGAIN, from the conversation and probably from the room. The actual exercise of excusing yourself from the conversation, going out and coming back is usually enough to break the cycle. Sometimes, you may need something better, try wrapping a towel around your head and screaming or punching a few pillows. You may just have time to do one of these things before they follow you and ask the same question again or demand that they want to go to the bank right now!

ARE THESE SCENARIOS FAMILIAR?

They can't remember what they had for lunch or even if they had lunch. However, if you just casually mentioned that you need to go to the bank they get that word in their mind and ask repeatedly if you can go now. Why they remember the one thing you don't want them to focus on is a question that we can't answer, so we just have to deal with it until we can get it changed. It is truly the time when we question if they really have an illness or if they are truly trying to drive us out of our minds and they are being successful.

In early stages, or early in the disease process, repetition is usually a serious problem, which creates chaos and discomfort. There are probably many reasons for this and the most logical is that they are trying to keep track of something when they are so aware that they can't really keep track of anything. They most often are fixated on finance and going somewhere. Thus the idea of leaving the house and talking finances takes on a high priority. This is truly a concern of responsibility for all of us, for we all need to know where we are, that we have a roof over our heads, and that we know how to pay the bills. If we don't, we understand disaster will occur. Consequently, they want to take care of these things but truly can't remember what has and hasn't been addressed, so they become very fixated.

Obviously, finances and items of a financial matter remain important to a person with AD. Therefore, if they can't find things especially of a financial nature then it is not paranoia for a person with AD to assume that someone has taken something. This concern, when combined with confusion and anxiety, can escalate to the point that the person truly believes someone has taken everything. This particularly applies to the things like money that are in the bank and cannot be seen.

Once again it seems important to digress somewhat to gain perspective on understanding this problem from a diagnostic point of view. By diagnosis, one has memory impairment resulting in the inability to learn new information or recall previously learned information. It stands to reason that the recent placement of things would be very likely to come under new information. When the person with AD can't recall the new information, then where he/she has just placed something will be a continuous mystery

Have you ever lost the car in a large shopping center? Isn't your initial reaction that it has been stolen? It seems quite natural to assume that it has been stolen rather than admit we were foolish, didn't pay attention, or have actually lost our car. Actually, it would almost be preferable for it to have been stolen! Have you ever lost your keys or a document that you need for a meeting in a few minutes? You feel foolish and frustrated and want someone else to blame. It is not likely that you could feel very good about yourself if this happened all of the time. Would it make sense to assume that you have intentionally hidden it from yourself? That would be the kind of logic a person with AD would need to adopt if they didn't accuse someone else of constantly taking their misplaced things.

The person with AD is still capable of tracking some things and not others and unfortunately there is truly little known rhyme or reason to this process. It is truly logical, for the person with AD, to focus on what is upsetting them.

65

They focus by asking the same questions over and over and by accusing others of misdeeds and then they become increasingly angry.

If our response is defensiveness and increased anger, then the problem increases on both sides. The negative downward spiral is in full swing and we are both lost. Since you, the caregiver, are also perfectly justified in your response, as it is so repetitive, then you need to find a way to REGROUP. The best method for this is to literally go out and come back in again - start over, do whatever it takes for you to regroup so you can effectively address the situation.

When you are no longer "losing it," then you can provide what they need most and that is reassurance that everything will be all right, that you will help them, and together you can do anything. This is not possible when you are "losing it".

Yes, I am referring to the same thing again, my simple list of Ten Absolutes and now, after you repeat and regroup, YOU, need to reassure them. One of the best ways of reassuring someone is to tell them that you will help and then show them you are with them by doing what they like and now you can enjoy each other by not being angry any longer. This is the time for diversion and distraction to their favorite things and when the situation calms down, you can laugh and smile again. Eventually, distraction and diversion should become the caregiver's favorite things. Once you are back in a calm state, then you can do whatever needs to be done. Probably you have spent less time than the arguments would have taken.

A caregiver shared her story of how this worked for her and it might be helpful for others. Her mother was truly beautiful, tiny, and looked very pristine and sweet. Actually, she had always had a very bad temper and was very volatile, though the family consistently hid and denied this fact. The little lady loved to go out and especially to lunch in restaurants. Her daughter very much wanted to spend time with her doing the things she loved. She took her to lunch one day at Denny's Restaurant near where she lived. The restaurant was unusually busy that day and the only available place to sit was in the front in a section with a lot of glass windows in a booth that was designed for a large group. They had a pleasant lunch and then she noticed her mother looking around probably for her purse. She could see that her mother was becoming upset and she knew that action needed to be taken quickly or the situation could become out of control and even volatile. She said that she suddenly remembered the instruction to regroup. So she excused herself, left the booth, went up to the front of the restaurant (only about 30 feet away) turned around and came back to the booth. She stopped by her mother and said "Hi, Mom, I am so happy to see you. Oh! You have already eaten. Well, will you at least let me buy you lunch? Let's go get some ice cream." Her mom, now pleasantly distracted, replied "O. K. honey." She got up and they happily proceeded to the cash register to pay the bill. As they were walking away the daughter looked back and the people in the area were all staring at her as if she were totally out of her mind. She laughingly reported that she really didn't care but she knew that they would have been very unhappy had she not regrouped. Instead of wondering about her mental status the observers could have been accused of stealing a purse and possibly even subjected to cursing, water being thrown on them, or something thrown at the window. She and her mother did go get ice cream, they had a very pleasant outing and she was never afraid to take her mother to lunch again.

MOST IMPORTANT!

How is it possible that they can get fixated on the one thing that they can't do? Why can't they get fixated on something you want them to do? Actually they can, but it will take work on your part to find what repetitive things they can do and will fixate on in order to eliminate their boredom and also to preserve your sanity.

This is truly one of the keys and it can be used. The reason you may need some help with this is because the things they always liked to do may be too difficult or too full of failure for them. In addition, what they can do may be too simple for you to design because it would bore you. Watch to see what they do, even if it drives you crazy, as it will be the strongest clue for what they can and will do repetitively to amuse themselves. This is the best way to create activities to prevent and alleviate boredom for them. If they like to load tools in the car, pack clothing for a trip, wash the dishes, or just take things from room to room. Turn this into an activity, encourage them to do what they do and provide them with things to do this with. If you keep them busy with their things then you will prevent their worries and you have reassured them. If you aren't yet successful with this then it is a project to work on - ask for help, especially from those who offer help and those who offer criticism. You might simply ask, "What would you do if you were me?" This is one of the best questions to alleviate your frustration and to actually get answers from someone that might accidentally be helpful.

If you will take the time to write down the repetitive behaviors I think you will be surprised, but probably shouldn't be, because the behaviors are very much the same and actually happen at about the same time every day. Once you know for certain that there is a pattern to behaviors, it will be easier for you to adjust and thus change the behaviors. Remember you can only change the situation by changing the environment to which they are trying to respond. The person with AD cannot change and you cannot change them. You can change yourself and ultimately if you get into the habit of analyzing the situation and changing how you react to it, you will change the environment and thus change the way the person with AD reacts. Everything will get better and easier and you can start enjoying each other again instead of "losing your mind".

NEVER SAY, "YOU CAN'T"

ALWAYS SHOW THEM WHAT THEY CAN DO

You can't:

"You can't wear two shirts, you can't pick that up with your hands, you can't eat that like that, you can't put your sweater on your legs, you can't put your shoe on your shoe, you can't go outside it is raining, you can't keep putting things in the wrong place, you can't go home you are home,"

You can:

"Try this one it looks nice, see how this spoon works, isn't this fun, try this on, try it over here, we need to find the umbrella, this looks nice here, I want to go home too."

NOW WHAT DOES THAT MEAN?

Do you remember when life seemed simple, when every task wasn't a struggle, when getting dressed was taken for granted? You really can go back to that time again but it will require, YOU GUESSED IT-ONCE AGAIN, that you make some changes in how YOU do things.

Many things that we do in the normal routine of life is habitual or by rote. If you are particularly stressed it is difficult to recall if you just did something or were going to do it and you become somewhat alarmed and say things like, "I must be losing my mind." or "What is wrong with me?" For example you usually take your vitamins right after your shower every morning, but one morning the phone rang as you got out of the shower and you went and answered the phone. You are now off the phone, have finished drying, have gotten dressed and are about ready to leave for the day and notice your vitamin bottle. Now you question yourself, "Did or didn't I take my vitamins when I came back from answering the phone." How do you feel as you are pondering this, are you able to retrace your actions in your mind? This is probably where persons with Alzheimer's Disease spend most of their time, in the wondering state. However they can only remain in that state very confused because they are unlikely to be able to retrace their steps. They continuously question did I or didn't I take my vitamins and then they are left with the feeling that something is missing, but they can't remember what it is. They just go back and forth trying to recall what it is that is missing.

Here are a couple of things that could happen to you when you are in this wondering state, choose which one would be most beneficial. If someone in your environment were to say:

"Do those vitamins leave an aftertaste? I saw you taking them with your orange juice this morning and I was wondering if it was to help with the taste or to swallow easier?"

"Why are you looking at your vitamins, I suppose you are trying to figure out if you've taken them again. Is there something wrong with you? You are doing that more and more; how can you possibly not be able to remember if you took your vitamins or not?"

With that in mind let's think about the simple things that a person with Alzheimer's Disease must do in the course of every day. If we can provide some direction and assistance rather than dismay and criticism, the person with Alzheimer's can focus on the task rather than their inadequacies.

It is important for you to remember that they may not be able to understand the words that you say but the tone you say them in comes through 'loud and clear'.

FAMILIAR SCENARIOS?
Inappropriate dressing:

Dressing inappropriately seems to be something that is left to individual taste. I don't care much about dressing as it takes too much time and I so often wish that we could just cover up and not worry about the rest. However, a person with Alzheimer's Disease really does get very confused with the task of dressing. It is not at all uncommon for them to wear very obvious inappropriate clothing. They may put on two shirts, two dresses, mismatched shoes and even more obvious and embarrassing things like having their underwear on the outside of their clothes.

Just imagine how it must feel to not even know how to get dressed anymore. How do you feel when you have put on something that you think looks fine and someone says, "You aren't going to wear that are you"? Now, how on earth is one to answer such a question? If you have something on and you are headed for the car of course that is what you intended to wear!!! However, after that comment it is obvious that you shouldn't wear it and your choices are to go and change or just be uncomfortable. Your defense is to want to strangle the person who uttered such an unnecessary statement.

I would suspect that the person with AD spends most of their time in this state of frustration and anger because the world constantly looks at them askance and reinforces with negative verbal terms that they have done yet another thing wrong. They can't keep track of what is wrong or what to do but they can keep track of the feeling that they are inadequate and you are reinforcing that inadequacy and you become the enemy.

If you will try to understand how this feels from their point of view it will be much easier to ONCE AGAIN - CHANGE YOU, because yes this continues to be how one deals with this disease process.

A positive change is to simply show them what they can do and for them getting dressed is a great start. Offer to be of assistance and hand them clothing in the order that they need to put on. Choice is a good thing and they will be very capable of refusing to wear something they don't want to wear. However, most of the time if you hand them things in order and use nonverbal cues, touch the leg or foot they need to use, they will concentrate on the process and not on the need to struggle.

For those who truly can't hold still long enough to get dressed in the correct order, you need to be even better organized and find a way to keep them in the general area so they won't appear in the wrong place in a state of undress. Placing a chair near the door that you can easily move in front of the doorknob is often a solution to their wandering out into the next room. Or if you will stand in front of the doorknob area and hand them things in the correct order, it too will help. If they are looking for a way out and you visually block the way out then they will circle around and come back to you for another try at what you are trying to accomplish. If they get away and go into an area that will create embarrassment and or frustration for both of you, then you will have a new set of problems.

MOST IMPORTANT!

In the beginning of this chapter a question was asked and is now repeated. Do you remember when life seemed simple, when every task wasn't a struggle, when getting dressed was taken for granted? You really can go back to that time again but it will require, YOU GUESSED IT-ONCE AGAIN, that you make some changes in how YOU do things.

A person with Alzheimer's Disease is painfully aware of how many things they can't do. If it is a struggle for those of us watching and trying to help, what must it feel like from the inside?

Assisting a person with Alzheimer's Disease with what they can do, rather than calling attention to their incompetence would seem obvious. However, if you stop and think about what you normally do, you will see that identifying their incompetence seems to come naturally.

You and all acquaintances should make it a project to focus on what the person with AD can do well. With this new focus you will be amazed at how easy it is to change negatives to positives.

The hidden benefit in this approach is that you soon begin to see your own success in task completion. You will get back to a life you had decided was lost. Struggles will diminish or disappear completely as you become more skilled. You will begin to feel that you once again have some control over your life. When small tasks like getting dressed stop being a struggle there is a distinct sense of well being. When you are in a state of well being other tasks become easier. It is very possible to return to an approach to life concentrating on things that make each day interesting. The most important part is that you can enjoy interactions with each other and accomplish what is important and not even attempt things that truly do not matter.

NEVER COMMAND/DEMAND

ALWAYS ASK/MODEL

Command/Demand:

"You have got to change your clothes, sit down right here and stop walking around, that doesn't belong to you now give it back, why would you take those we didn't pay for them, you have to leave your clothes on you are in a public restroom, we are in a hurry you need to do this right now."

Ask/Model:

"This is pretty, do you want to try it on, sit with me a minute (pat the chair), this is nice may I see it, do you want to buy those, see if you will be warmer with this, how about going here."

NOW WHAT DOES THAT MEAN?

When we have the continuous responsibility of looking out for someone who is becoming more disabled in the areas we all take for granted such as planning and sequencing, it becomes very frustrating to accomplish tasks. This is complicated if we are going to insist that they do things the way they have always done them, or if we insist that they can do nothing for themselves, and we need to do it for them, because we are in a hurry. It is human nature for our emotions to escalate when becoming frustrated and it shows quickly in action and words. Especially when you have an appointment or have company coming or have something that needs to be done within a specific time frame, you can count on TROUBLE!

What is actually happening here is that you

are becoming commanding and demanding and they are responding exactly the same way to you. You are insisting on what you want and they are insisting that they don't want it. There is an easy lesson in this and it is to ONCE AGAIN - CHANGE YOU. You can use their image of you to your advantage but first you need to calm down, focus on what you are trying to accomplish and show them what to do.

If you are in trouble already then it is too late to ask or expect cooperation, but it is not too late to model for them as to what to do. I am not suggesting that you need to take off your clothes and show them how to get undressed. It is actually much less complicated than that. If you want them to lift a leg, then lift yours or touch theirs and it will happen almost magically. This modifying technique is certainly better than trying to yell them into lifting a leg.

Though there are all kinds of studies about mirror imaging, I really hadn't originally thought to use it with persons with Alzheimer's Disease. The way I discovered that this worked was through a perfectly worn out cowardly act of trying to disappear when I couldn't deal for one more second with the ravages of Alzheimer's Disease on one of the patients.

ARE THESE SCENARIOS FAMILIAR?
Getting in and out of the car:

I had spent one of those 4-hour stints that seemed like 24 in the doctor's office with a little lady with Alzheimer's Disease. Now I am sure you would agree that a book needs to be written on how to get through any medical appointment without disaster and exhaustion but we will postpone that idea for now.

We, my little lady patient and I, had finally finished; we had made it through the Dr. appointment and had finally gotten into the elevator and out to the car to GO HOME! We were both exhausted and so DONE with the entire day. We got to the car, opened the door and you GUESSED IT, RIGIDITY SET IN. She was truly the cutest, little, sweet, grandmother-looking-lady you have ever seen. White hair in a bun, little glasses, round loving cheeks and so dainty and helpless. She had one leg in the car, the other on the ground, one hand on the top of the door opening, the other on the door and her arms and legs became locked in a state of rigidity. If you have experienced this scenario you know that this frozen state is nearly impossible to change. She apparently became frightened as I was trying in vain to get some body part, like a hand or a leg, to release so we could get into the car. She leaned out her sweet little head and began to pitifully yell, "Help, Help, I am being taken to be killed". I just have to admit that I knew I would soon be in jail and the only thing I could think to do in my overtaxed state was to hide. I literally ducked behind her, sat down in her seat, and she sat on top of me, which released the rigidity. I was able to slide out from under and get her to move her other leg into the car and we went HOME! I realized that what I had done was modeling what she should do and surprisingly she did it. Now I know that it isn't really hiding but modeling!! See, every once in awhile when working with this disease process, we get a break. We serendipitously come across something that works when we have absolutely given up!

Eating:

Modeling can be very helpful in the dining room or in a restaurant when the person with Alzheimer's Disease becomes rigid and just can't sit down. If you will get them to look at you and then model that you are sitting down they will do the same. It truly seems to be individual as to whether a booth or a table is preferable in a restaurant. If you are trying to sit in a booth and they can't sit down, try sitting on the opposite side as a demonstration. If that doesn't work get them to turn the direction of the booth, walk behind them as close as you can get so they feel you and then sit down right beside them, they are likely to follow you into the booth. The table seems easier initially as it is easier to demonstrate how to sit. However, tables are often in the middle and there is more distraction and confusion from that angle and they may be less able to sit comfortably for the period of time that a meal takes. If at all possible take them to the restaurants they have always frequented and sit where you have always sat.

Very often weight loss becomes a big problem as the person with Alzheimer's Disease forgets to eat, becomes too distracted to eat or simply can't perform the mechanics of eating. The logical response is to try to feed them. However, this response almost always results in refusal to eat and increases the weight loss problem. There are a few individuals with AD that eat only when fed and this should be the last resort not the first one. Feeding someone takes a lot of time and energy and it removes a level of independence, for the person with AD, that is likely to be essential for their mental well being. Feeding someone is creating a 'lose-lose proposition'.

Modeling and altering caregiver expectations are two key items to eliminating the weight loss problem. Modeling is easy in this instance as you can effectively model by eating with them, preferably sitting across from them. Altering expectations is more difficult because it means one more step in accepting that the disease is progressing; it is not going to go away.

Telling them they must eat and reminding them to hurry and verbally encouraging them goes back to almost all of the absolutes. You are reasoning, lecturing, shaming, showing them what they can't do and ultimately probably even arguing. This is obviously not the best atmosphere for a positive dining experience.

A very pleasant social experience in our society is to share a meal or dessert at a table with someone we care about. This is evidenced in social language with, "Let's meet for a drink, let's do lunch, can you come by for coffee, we always had a big Sunday dinner for the entire family". You can use this socially acceptable practice to enhance eating and eating pleasure; it is simple and it gives you some rest. Focus on a pleasant experience; do not focus on making them eat. I ask, "Do you or anyone you know, want to do something someone is trying to make you do? Don't you automatically become resistive?"

Using modeling with eating is truly simple. Just sit across from them wherever possible and share a meal. They can see what you are doing and they can do the same. What if you are in a professional care situation where you are not allowed to eat with the person with AD or if you are not hungry or you have finished eating? The answer is to pretend! Always sit down, in their visual plane and go through the motions of eating, using a utensil makes it easier and more realistic - you do not have to have food in the utensil to model.

What if they are having difficulty with the mechanics of eating? Some of the more common problems are:

- Not getting food on the fork
- Pushing food off of the plate
- Eating in a pattern (only in the center of the plate or on one side)
- Pouring or mixing food
- Picking things up inappropriately with utensils
- Picking things up inappropriately with fingers
- Rearranging dishes and utensils
- Eating the paper napkin.

This is the area where the caregiver must alter expectations and it is important to be creative and provide them with assistance. The goal is to make sure they eat. The creativity is in finding ways for them to eat with no embarrassment, minimal assistance and independence.

The most obvious and successful for addressing the issues mentioned in the last paragraph are as follows:

If there are problems getting food on the fork, trade it for a spoon. Next time start with a spoon and remove the fork from their visual area.

If food is sliding off of the plate start using a plate with a lip or place their food in a bowl that matches the other dishes. Avoid dishes that are obviously adapted such as the stainless steel plate guard, etc.

If they are eating in a pattern they are having visual problems. Discreetly reach over and turn the plate so they can see the other sections.

If they are pouring and mixing food then start serving them restaurant style with one item at a time, this includes beverages.

If they are picking up things inappropriately with utensils, for example they are trying to pick up the dinner roll with a fork. Place finger foods on another plate at the side and encourage them to eat that next.

If they are picking up things inappropriately with their fingers, it is time to switch to finger foods. Substitute roast beef with a roast beef sandwich, mashed potatoes with french fries, salad with fresh fruits and vegetables, soft desserts in an ice cream cone. This is also an excellent method for encouraging persons with AD who are unable to sit still at the table to eat. Provide them with finger foods that they can eat 'on the go' each time they approach the table.

If they are rearranging the dishes and utensils remove the distractions from their visual plane. Use a single colored placemat with one dish and one eating utensil, if they eat mostly finger foods you may need to move the eating utensil and hand it to them only when they need it.

Sometimes they can no longer discern what is edible. This is often evidenced with their attempts at eating the paper napkin or shredding it and placing the shreds in their food. Replace the paper napkin with a cloth one; you may then need to place the cloth napkin out of their sight and offer it only when needed.

Two final and important dining tips are: First, use modeling to get them to wipe their faces, especially around their mouths when eating. If you motion to their napkin and then wipe your mouth where theirs needs to be wiped, they can eat without unnecessary mess or embarrassment. Second, finish the meal by providing them with warm washcloths (sort of an expansion of the finger bowl), and motion for them to wash their faces. This is so much more dignified than washing their faces for them at the table. It is also very pleasant to finish a meal with warm washcloths it makes one feel pampered rather than inept. Wet washcloths can be warmed in the microwave if running warm water is inconvenient.

Toileting:

One of the most useful places that modeling can be effective is in toileting, a subject that most caregivers hate. One of the main reasons for family members finally giving up on trying to care for a person with AD is when he/she doesn't remember the mechanics of toileting. This is an area of concern poorly addressed in most professional care settings.

There is a simple sound solution to the

problem of urinating and defecating in improper places and having to clean someone up who has had an accident, even in disposable undergarments. Men tend to urinate in yards, closets and corners, creating embarrassment and persistent smells in the environment. Women use wastebaskets and closet floors, and consistently flush soiled undergarments. Both men and women way too often suffer the loss of dignity by soiling themselves 'to add insult to injury'. They then have to fight someone who is trying to remove their soiled clothing. They do not understand the purpose is to wash their skin to prevent smell and skin breakdown. They just know they are uncomfortable and embarrassed and now someone wants them to remove their underwear! If a person with AD is taken to the toilet regularly and they have eliminated waste in the toilet, then they will not eliminate waste inappropriately; therefore a huge problem will be solved.

There are those of us who truly believe that toileting solves this problem of urinating and defecating in inappropriate places. The difficulty is in getting caregivers to buy into this thought pattern. First, a caregiver must agree to monitor a routine for toileting and second, they have to have enough of a rapport with the person with AD to allow them to take them to the toilet. Initially, the process becomes experimental, as their toileting pattern must be assessed. This is done by trial and error. It is thought that people in general only urinate about every two hours. This is a good place to start, take them to the toilet every two hours. If they are dry and they use the toilet, then you can stick with every two hours. If they are already wet then you need to shorten the time to take them. Try in 1 hour and forty-five minutes. Keep track of the times they really go and that will become their routine for toileting.

When you are toileting a person with AD regularly a frustrating and commonplace situation can occur. Sometimes when you get them in the bathroom, they actually let you assist with the removal of their undergarments, they get to the toilet, and rigidity sets in again. They cannot seem to sit down on the toilet. We try pushing on their shoulders, touching the back of their knees etc. to no avail. It is not at all unusual that, because they are in the bathroom with undergarments down, they will often urinate while standing up in front of the toilet, which is embarrassing and frustrating for all. If you can get beside them and get them to look at you and you sit down or squat, almost always they will sit down too and then you just have to get them on track as to why they are sitting on the toilet! This works for men also and I have just accepted the fact that I will probably have to toilet men by having them sit down. I can't find a way to demonstrate how to toilet standing and since the majority of caregivers seem to be women this seems to be one of the main reasons that men aren't toileted routinely.

MOST IMPORTANT!

Often what we are trying to get them to do just doesn't make sense to them. We get frustrated and try to use language to get them to respond. When that doesn't work and it rarely does, we become more demanding and we become frustrated. Increasingly, our frustration shows in our use of language and also in the strong nonverbal cues to which they quickly respond with refusal, belligerence and even aggressiveness. We are once again on that never ending road to nowhere that results in tears and frustration and we feel the need to just QUIT.

I am suggesting a very simple solution and it works for as many things that you are willing to try it with. It is often so simple and works so well that even the most seasoned caregivers forget to use it. The person with AD will almost always truly model or do exactly what you show them to do. Use large muscle movements like dressing, sitting, standing and the smaller ones like eating or drinking. This is such a simple solution and for once requires VERY LITTLE CHANGING ON YOUR PART, which by now must be quite welcome. The payoff is that you will become more and more successful at completing tasks and doing things in a timely manner. It requires merely developing consistency in using modeling, with a smile and thank you when completed. THE RULE IS TO TALK LESS AND SHOW MORE. By doing so, you will reap the rewards of success in the areas that you have learned to dread and avoid.

NEVER CONDESCEND

ALWAYS ENCOURAGE/PRAISE

Never Condescend:
"Did you have any problems with him today. Be
sure he takes his medicine; he spit it out this morning.
I hope you don't have trouble today it took me 20
minutes just to get him into the car. He has been
looking for his mother all morning."
Always Encourage/Praise
"I'm sure you were your sweet wonderful self today.
Dad will help you with his medicine today, it has been
hard to swallow. We are having a challenging day
today and dad will help you a lot, he is especially
interested in his mother today."

NOW WHAT DOES THAT MEAN?

There was a time in the not too distant past
where we actually talked to a person with A D as if
they were deaf and probably Developmentally
Disabled. There were several reasons for this
approach. The early teachings for working with a
person with AD emphasized the plaques and
tangles. It was explained that because the
messages in the brain were interrupted by the
plaques and tangles it was important to speak
slowly as it took longer for them to process the
messages. Dealing with older people seemed to
hold a natural assumption that if you were old you
were hard of hearing. Consequently, very well
intentioned persons would get right close to a
person with AD and speaking very loudly and very
slowly say something like, "DO YOU WANT TO

COME WITH ME?" The response to this was that the person with AD was likely to hit you right in the mouth or at least push you away. When we first encouraged caregivers not to condescend, this was the first area to correct. Fortunately, we have progressed way beyond that approach so it is no longer a problem.

What is a problem is that we continue to talk about a person with AD in front of them as if they aren't even there. This is very condescending and we are not doing it to be unkind and certainly not to make them angry or upset. The main reason we do this is to provide instruction and information. This is almost always done at the time when they are being left by the caregiver or there is a shift change in a care setting. Then the caretaker insists that the reason they had problems with the person with AD was they were angry for being left or they were sundowning. Sundowning is a common term for the evening hours when it has been proclaimed that persons with AD have the most difficult time of their day.

I would like to propose that the person with AD is angry because they were being talked about in front of them as if they were invisible. They feel they aren't important and don't matter. Even if they don't understand what is being said they do understand that they are being talked about. Remember, it is natural to assume that if you are being talked about it is usually in the negative. This can hurt their feelings and even if they repress it at the time, may still act out on those hurt feelings later on.

Giving instructions is important and it is

essential for the caregiver to both give instructions and also to inquire about what has happened during the day/night. It is also therapeutic for the caregiver to be able to vent to a sympathetic person. So how do we accomplish a flow of important information without talking about the person with AD in front of them? When and how can you find the opportunity to vent, especially if you have had a bad day?

It is really simple. Write the instructions. Writing everything down is the best method of communication and it is an accurate reference after you are gone. If there is something that just happened and isn't included on the instructions then incorporate this information into the conversation.

For example, put your arm around the person with AD so he is incorporated in the conversation and you both speak together to the person who is providing instruction or relaying information. Say (use the AD person's name), Jim and I have been having 'a Monday' today we couldn't get any medicine to taste good enough to swallow. The car wouldn't cooperate, we had a terrible time getting in. Jim can't find his mother so will you please help him. We are both about ready to give up or start over."

This imparts the information without talking about him; instead you are talking with him as a part of the conversation. The tone of voice you use, the nonverbal cues such as holding hands or putting an arm around him makes him feel loved and included. Helping him to feel loved and included eliminates or reduces the frustration and hurt feelings that may have been experienced with the struggles.

It is human to ask questions about how things went and this is something that is of particular interest for the primary caregiver. The caregivers often feel guilty for having left the person with AD and they want reassurance that it was fine. On the other hand the caregiver is fearful that if the person with AD did just fine without the caregiver then the caregiver won't be needed any longer. If the report is bad and the person with AD did not do well, the caregiver is needed but feels guilty that they left the person with AD and created unhappiness. For the caregiver this is a lose-lose cycle and this is the very reason that outside assistance is necessary for a successful journey through this disease process. Support Groups are free, available and very necessary. Ultimately, questions will be asked by the caregiver, in front of the person with AD which need to be answered. They should be answered in the same manner as just previously discussed. Include the person with AD in the conversation physically with touch and talk to the person asking questions as if you and the person with AD are answering together. This seems little and petty but makes an incredible difference in the consistency of their being content and comfortable especially in new situations.

ARE THESE SCENARIOS FAMILIAR?

In the six years that I took care of Helen H. we never learned why she always started out each of my visits so angry. We assumed that it was because her daughters usually left right after I arrived. She would be very angry and try to hurt me the minute they left. I have to admit that we all accepted her behavior as a part of the disease. However, after I had Helen N. living with me I found that she would do very much the same thing when I left her and she certainly didn't see me as her daughter. I was another caregiver. I had also noted that she wouldn't wake up angry but was only angry when she saw me leave or so I thought. Then one day I happened to notice that she was standing back with her hand by her face as if she were whispering to someone and pointing to the relief caregiver and myself. I saw it as a revelation that she perceived us as talking about her and we were. I immediately changed and we saw an amazing decline in her reaction to the relief caregivers. I then tried the same approach on Helen H. and believed that it made a difference. However, by that stage she was much less aware of what was going on and had reduced her reactions to me. Until then we had believed that she had become accustomed to my approaches and also that she was just not as aware of her environment.

Though we didn't do an empirical study to prove the results there is a definite pattern. If we do not make them angry by talking about them, their time with a substitute caregiver is much more pleasant and starts off much better.

MOST IMPORTANT!
Just as with all of the information being provided in this book this is not a tip that should be used to make you feel guilty. If you now realize that you have been talking about a person with AD

in front of them for whatever reason, to give instructions, or to get someone else to understand that indeed there is something wrong. Do not waste time and energy worrying about yesterday as you can't change it anyway. Use the information to become more determined to be aware of this as a problem and work on changing - YES ONCE AGAIN YOU HAVE TO CHANGE - your approach. There are even payoffs with the change you will have to make, your efforts will provide better visits and ultimately provide you with the opportunity to leave them more often, thus you will be taking better care of yourself.

It is not mentioned nearly often enough but the thing that is most important to your loved one with AD is that you continue to be available to look out for their needs. This does not mean you are the only one that can provide their care. The 36 Hour Day was aptly named because it takes 36 hours a day to keep up with a person that is cognitively impaired. It is virtually impossible for someone to do this successfully over a long period of time without it adversely affecting his or her life and health. If you overwork, without appropriate rest and leisure you will become ill and could even die. This would be the worst thing for every one concerned; the person with AD will not have someone to take care of their best interests which is what they need the most.

People say that they will do anything to make sure the person with AD is cared for at home. This heroic way of thinking may be placing themselves and ultimately the person with AD at risk. In addition, this situation often includes the services of a sitter. Often, a sitter and the person with AD do not have anything in common. In a situation where the person with AD spends their time with persons with whom they never had anything in common it is logical for them to be bored and feel useless which can contribute to unnecessary behavior problems and depression. This too is a lose-lose situation based on the best of intentions.

ABSOLUTELY NEVER FORCE

ALWAYS REINFORCE

<u>Force:</u>
"Now you are going to take a bath because you haven't had one for two weeks. These nice people are here to help us. Give that to me right now it is not yours. If you don't give it back we will have to take it from you. You may not go into this room, you must come out of this room right now"
<u>Reinforce:</u>
"I know you already took a bath, come right in here, I know you don't want a bath, lets take off this shoe. I know you don't want a bath, this lady is helping, and it will be O.K. That is really pretty, may I see it. Do you like this, would you like to have it? Isn't this a pretty room, would you like to go have a cup of coffee."

NOW WHAT DOES THAT MEAN?

In this disease process it is truly amazing how important unimportant things become. The bath is one of the biggest problems. For some reason that no one seems to understand, it is very difficult for a person with AD to let a family member or anyone to undress him or her and give them a bath. Yet not one of us would be comfortable letting someone take off our clothing and give us a bath. We really need to understand that this is indeed difficult and we need to act accordingly.

First of all the idea that they need a bath every day probably needs to be rethought. Taking a bath every day is not particularly good for the skin and it is not a habit that the majority of these persons had in their early life. For all real purposes the regressive part of this disease has the person with AD back in that early part of life.

Focus on the end result; they need to be clean. How that is accomplished should not be the focus. Bathing needs to be for a purpose, not a routine and it needs to be done with care.

I can't tell you how often the subject of bathing comes up and families tell me that this was when the person with AD reached the combative stage of their disease. Others will say that it took 5 people to just give a bath. Many care settings, before they learned that it didn't work, would have several people force a person with AD to take a bath on the night shift so no one would hear the screaming.

I believe that I can bring any reader of this book to the combative stage, by doing to them exactly what is done to a person with AD. We absolutely must think through what we are doing and why. They are not in the combative stage of their disease as much as they are reacting to what is being done to them. This would be normal for any frightened human. They can become unusually strong in these situations and that is not their disease; it is a response called fight or flight. It is self-defense, it is not Alzheimer's Disease.

ARE THESE SCENARIOS FAMILIAR?

Taking a bath:

It appears that I have told you what not to do-NEVER FORCE - but what do you do instead REINFORCE. Initially, a very acceptable reaction would be that the author of the book just doesn't understand this situation, but actually, because it is such a consistent area of difficulty it has become the specialty of this author. What follows will be several detailed scenarios describing exactly what to do and how to do it to perform the bath, when it must be done completely and when it needs to be done routinely.

When the bath must be done completely and immediately (Emergency):

Let's suppose that someone has had an accident and has soiled himself or herself with Diarrhea. Now, of course that has to be taken care of and certainly as soon as possible especially for their own good. No one wants to remain soiled and not only is there a smell but the furniture and floor will be damaged, perhaps beyond repair, if something isn't done immediately.

There is no disagreement here; something must be done immediately. However, what you need to do immediately is realize how frightening and embarrassing this is for the person with AD and everyone reacting is very detrimental. Let us digress for a moment to provide the opportunity of getting in touch with what the person with AD might be feeling. Have you ever fallen down? Isn't the first thing you do, even before you decide if you are hurt, is look around to see if anyone saw you fall? Why do you do that? Isn't it because it is embarrassing and you want to see who has witnessed that embarrassment, you hope no one saw don't you? If someone did see and they offer to help don't you just want to become invisible, to have them go away? Well, falling is a simple thing,

99

falling happens to everyone. Just imagine, if you can, how much more embarrassing it would be to have soiled yourself? Then imagine if it is in public, at a dinner or even in the home. Suppose that the response is the look of repulsion on every face. Everyone reacts immediately, and you, the person with AD become the center of negative attention.

If you can identify with what they are feeling then you will agree the steps to solve this problem are not only practical, they are kind and considerate. The first thing you need to do is befriend the person with AD, and discreetly ask others to leave the room. If it is in a large care facility, in a common area, then encourage staff to move everyone to a different part of the room. What you are creating is a less embarrassing environment. Next, get something large and washable, a sheet is an excellent item and usually readily available. Use this sheet to wrap around them, it is best to suggest that they must be cold and wrap it from their shoulders, be cautious that you don't leave something for them to trip on. This shows that you want to help and don't think they are offensive. Then give them a few moments to regain their composure. You can busy yourself in the immediate area by covering things (such as furniture etc. that could be soiled) with washable material, like a few more sheets. Then if the person with AD does sit down in the wrong place it need not be permanently soiled. If you have someone else available to help, then suggest they get things ready such as a change of clothing and warm water in the bath or shower. If you don't have anyone available then suggest that the person with AD sit down and relax and go get things ready yourself. Definitely do not have several people standing around talking and wondering what to do; act as if nothing is happening.

Now that some time has passed and this only needs to be five minutes, you are ready to address the situation. Befriend them in order to get them to come with you. You may need to offer them a cup of coffee or hot chocolate or something to completely distract them from the situation. While this might sound gross, it is often very effective. When they seem calm and you have developed a friendly helpful rapport ask them to come with you, take them with you and lead toward the place for cleaning them up. When you get into the bathroom, if they are still reluctant to disrobe, get them into the shower area with their clothing on. You can almost always get their shoes off and the way you do this is something like the following, "I know you don't want a bath, sit right here (preferably on the shower stool) please lift this foot, perfect, slide that right off, perfect, thank you, now the other one, I know you took a bath yesterday, is this water nice and warm (run it on their hand only), doesn't it feel good?" If you can get beyond removing the shoes to take off the soiled garments, wonderful. However, you may have to be satisfied with only removing the shoes. In this complex situation you just need to think of what you are trying to accomplish, which is removing the diarrhea from them and from the clothing. The clothing will need to be rinsed anyway and what better spot than in the shower or tub. If the person with AD is still reluctant to remove their clothing, quickly and efficiently without appearing to rush, wet the clothing with warm water. Then apologize that they are all wet and help them remove the wet clothing. While they are concentrating on removing it with your assistance, you continue to wash off their body with the warm water. If you haven't done this before it does require skill and you will have to just learn to expect to get yourself wet. The goal at this stage is twofold, getting the soiled clothing off and getting the diarrhea off of their bodies. Have plenty of warm towels and a couple of soapy washcloths ready in advance. Hand them a soapy washcloth, if their hands are holding something they will be less likely to grab for the shower wand or hit. Point to areas that need to be washed and while they are washing you can assist with your own soapy washcloth. This needs to be done quickly and efficiently and your next goal is to get them as clean as possible and get them out. It is helpful to sincerely provide reinforcement and reassurance, "Let me help with that, wash right here, that is excellent, thank you for helping me, let's hurry and get out, whew! I finally got that water off, here this towel will be warm, let me help you dry, step right out here, sit down here, let's put this on, that is just perfect, thank you for helping me, etc." There is a fine balance between talking too much and not talking at all; it really depends on the person and you have to be able to determine what is working best with each individual. Ultimately, and always, it is your tone, your concern, and your desire to help them, which will create success. Don't use force. Don't linger and don't go for perfection, this is not the time to wash hair or concentrate on toenails. You are getting the diarrhea off, making sure they are comfortable, and completing the process quickly. The secondary bonus in this process is that the clothing will be almost completely rinsed and ready for the washer as the bath is completed. Lead them away from the bath area to do something they like and enjoy so the 'good feelings get going.' If you are their hero then stay with them for the good things. If they are angry with you then turn them over to someone else who will change the subject to good things. If you are alone and they are angry with you, quickly give them something they like, in a safe place and leave the room to go and clean up the rest of the mess. In a few minutes (at least 5, 10 for higher functioning person) you can return and behave as if you have just arrived for the day. Greet them warmly and offer something they like. There are few blessings to forgetfulness but in this disease process if you will forget that they are angry with you and they will too. Regroup, start over, make friends, enjoy each other. Don't bring up the past with items such as, "Are you still angry with me?"

This entire process provides reinforcement, avoids force, and takes care of a very messy and potentially volatile situation. It prevents damage and honestly takes less time than a battle. The ultimate reward is that no one gets hurt and you may never have to see the "combative stage of his or her disease".

When the bath must be done routinely:

The previous process generally works for most bathing situations. However, there will be times when you cannot get them into the bathroom, especially for routine care. If you cannot get them into the bathroom, use towels and sheets to cover the bed, floor, and a chair in the bedroom. Bring in a plastic pan of warm soapy washcloths, a stack of dry washcloths, and two small plastic pans of warm water. A nailbrush is useful in one of the pans of water. Start by washing their hands by putting their hands in the water and using the nailbrush. Then wash their face, hand them a washcloth and model what to do. Have them assist you in taking off their shoes and soaking their feet and assist them in drying their feet. Change their shirt/blouse and wipe off underarm area. Always give them a washcloth and move their hands to the place you want them to start, and surprisingly they will almost always wash themselves. Do the lower area last, hand them two rags so each of their hands are busy when you assist them with pulling down their pants and underwear. If they become angry, stop, change the subject, agree with them and start again. If you are sensing too much anger then stop, consider the job partially done. Go get a clean pan of water or a cup of coffee, etc. and come back and try again. You may need to be satisfied with only part of a bath in the a.m. and more in the p.m. If you are unsuccessful in getting to the pubic area with the partial bath you can do it next time they are in the bathroom. Keep your bathrooms well stocked with towels, washcloths, disposable undergarments and at least one complete change of clothing for the person with AD. When they are on the toilet offer them a warm soapy cloth to "wash up", assist them quickly and efficiently from the rear, when they stand up. If you cannot touch or they won't use the cloth, get small plastic bottles (squirt not spray ends) and fill with warm soapy water and quickly squirt over the perineal area into the toilet. This isn't perfect but goes a long way towards accomplishing the ultimate goal of keeping them clean and odor free.

When they insist on taking things that are not theirs:

Initially, assess how important the issue really is. They will often just put it down in a few minutes anyway. However, if it is an issue with someone else and is causing a lot of distress for others or for the environment then trade for something they like. Do not forcefully take anything away even if it is unsafe. Quickly and efficiently negotiate a trade for something else. This really is a simple process and will be accomplished easily if you don't insist on creating an argument or a battle of the wills. If you get into a battle of the wills, wait 5 minutes and then try with something new to trade. Be patient and kind and spend your time talking to the person who is upset with the person with AD. Trying to reason with the person with AD does not work.

If they insist on going into places where they are not welcome:

Please assess how important this issue really is. If it is in your own home, be sure to have places where they can go and have the freedom to touch and rearrange everything. Do invest in placing items under lock and key or in glass showcases so they will be safe and not so inviting.

This is usually an issue in long-term care

situations when the person with AD is wandering. Initially, if someone is wandering they are probably bored and need something interesting to do. Invite them pleasantly to come with you to do something interesting. Do not tell them that they shouldn't be where they are, or scold them, or try to force them to go somewhere else. Greet them as if you had been searching for them and ask them to join you in going to a new place. Drop the subject and do not waste your time or their energy trying to make them understand that they can't do something or go somewhere again.

If the person whose room they have been in is angry, and they do not have a dementia diagnosis, tell them you will be back later to discuss plans with them and leave the area. If the person whose room they have been in does have a dementia diagnosis then getting out of sight will be automatically out of mind and will solve the problem. Do not bring up issues once they are past, leave them in the area of recent things which they can't remember or keep track.

MOST IMPORTANT!

The reason a person with AD has to be forced to do anything is based mainly on our need and not related to their need. We are afraid that they are dirty and offensive and will soil our homes and that is important. They get into things that belong to others and we don't want them to get into trouble and we don't want to be embarrassed. This isn't just about our embarrassment it is about knowing they too would have been embarrassed if they knew they were doing these things that seem so inappropriate. I am not suggesting that the motivation for demanding control of their actions is selfish. It is just misunderstood. Remember that some of their actions are not really as important as they seem. Stop and think, "Is this an emergency? Is it life threatening?" If the answer is no then relax and think of a new approach that accomplishes the task without force.

Relaxing about the things that are usually handled with force will take some serious rethinking and some serious practice. The questions need to be continuously asked, "How important is it and what will happen if it has to wait?" If it is not truly life threatening then it can wait or be skipped altogether and the combative, aggressive, catastrophic reaction part of the disease can be eliminated in all stages.

THE BEGINNING

HOPE

Now that you have finished this book I hope you can think of it as the beginning and not the end. Are you ever going to become perfect at this? I think not. Is anything in life or in any relationship perfect? But you can become trained and relaxed and those two items will make everything much better. Will there be days when you just can't cope with this? Absolutely, and on those days the very best thing for both of you is for you to go somewhere else at least for a period of time. It is essential, probably more for the person with AD than for the caregiver that you begin immediately to find someone that can stay with the person with AD and or get them into a day care situation. You are already behind if you have not done this and you need to do it TODAY - do not wait. Thinking that you are the only one that should be with them is not in their best interest or in yours and you MUST change that thinking if you don't adopt anything else in this book.

They need a break from you as much as or maybe even more than you need a break from them. It is not good for either of you to live in a constant state of frustration and burn out. Please call your local Alzheimer's Association for resource guidance and ask your family and friends to assist. If people are reluctant to help it is because they do not know what to do or how to do it. You need to tell them what you need and provide them with the tools for success. Call them on the phone and tell them that you need them to come and stay a few hours and give them some basic instructions. Then above all do not criticize or question what they have done - appreciate it and show your appreciation with a smile and a thank you.

NOW WHAT DOES THAT MEAN?

It is a natural part of your grief process over the loss of the person you once knew that causes you to be protective and critical. This scares off most of your assistance and you need to be aware that you are creating a nightmare for yourself and for the person with AD you are creating isolation. Everyone needs to have friends and other people in their lives and you need to get away for a bath, a movie, a haircut, to shop for groceries or just to go to the bathroom uninterrupted. If you will practice accepting help and allowing others to work through their difficulties facing the Alzheimer's Disease process, everyone will be better and happier and this journey doesn't have to be so lonely and hopeless for you. There is help and there is hope. Is it perfect? Absolutely not! But it is there and you just need to learn how to find and accept it. Finding help and hope is the last CHANGE that you must make but it is the most important so it should be the FIRST chapter of the book. It is the FIRST thing you need to do and tomorrow is too late, do it today. You, the caregiver, will feel better and so will the person with AD. If you feel guilty that you aren't doing everything as I suggested, be kind to yourself and give the new processes time. The theme of this chapter is to start getting help today and that process is lengthy but IT CANNOT WAIT. You must ask for help and you must use help. YOU CANNOT DO THIS ALONE. If you can't get the help for free, then do whatever it takes to pay for assistance but get assistance immediately. If the first assistance you get isn't what you want, then keep trying. If at first you don't succeed try and try and try again but do not try to take care of a person with Alzheimer's Disease without assistance.

Last but certainly not least when working with a person with AD you need to TRY to Never: argue, reason, shame, lecture, say "remember", say "I Told You", say "you can't", command, demand or force. But if you find yourself doing these things, AND YOU WILL, then don't despair. What you need to do instead is just switch to the right side of the Ten Absolutes list and agree, divert, distract, reassure, reminisce, repeat, regroup, show them what they can do, ask, model, and reinforce. There is no magic formula, the items are all interchangeable but they do work and they will make life easier for the caregiver and the person with Alzheimer's Disease.

TEN ABSOLUTES
ABSOLUTELY NEVER!!!!!!!!!!!!!!!

1. ARGUE	instead	AGREE
2. REASON	instead	DIVERT
3. SHAME	instead	DISTRACT
4. LECTURE	instead	REASSURE
5. SAY "REMEMBER"	instead	REMINISCE
6. SAY "I TOLD YOU"	instead	REPEAT/REGROUP
7. SAY "YOU CAN'T"	instead	DO WHAT THEY CAN
8. COMMAND/DEMAND	instead	ASK/MODEL
9. CONDESCEND	instead	ENCOURAGE/PRAISE
10. FORCE	instead	REINFORCE

ABOUT THE AUTHOR

Jo Huey worked with persons with Alzheimer's Disease or a related disorder in 24 hour care settings from 1986 thru the Hurricane Katrina evacuation in 2005. She currently provides messages of help and hope to caregivers through presentations across the United States. She has a Certificate in Gerontology from the University of Denver and a Master of Social Science from the University of Colorado where her thesis was "Effectiveness of Training for Alzheimer's Caregivers." She lives in Colorado and New Orleans. She has two grown children, a daughter and son, and three grandsons.